Can We Say

NO?

Can We Say NO?

The Challenge of Rationing Health Care

Henry J. Aaron *and* William B. Schwartz

with Melissa Cox

BROOKINGS INSTITUTION PRESS
Washington, D.C.

Library of Congress Cataloging-in-Publication data

Aaron, Henry J.
   Can we say no? : the challenge of rationing health care / Henry J. Aaron and
William B. Schwartz ; with Melissa A. Cox.
      p.   cm.
   Includes bibliographical references and index.
   Summary: "Examines the use of rationing as a means to curb health care
spending, using the experience of Great Britain to highlight the promises and
pitfalls of this approach"—Provided by publisher.
   ISBN-13: 978-0-8157-0120-0 (cloth : alk. paper)
   ISBN-10: 0-8157-0120-9 (cloth : alk. paper)
   ISBN-13: 978-0-8157-0121-7 (pbk. : alk. paper)
   ISBN-10: 0-8157-0121-7 (pbk. : alk. paper)
   1. Health care rationing—Great Britain. 2. Health care rationing—United States.
3. Medical care, Cost of—Great Britain. 4. Medical care, Cost of—United States.
I. Schwartz, William B., 1922–   . II. Title.
   [DNLM: 1. Health Care Rationing—Great Britain. 2. Health Care Rationing—
United States. 3. Health Expenditures—Great Britain. 4. Health Expenditures—
United States. WA 540 FA1 A113c 2005]
   RA410.5.A23 2005
   362.1'0425—dc22   2005024433

9 8 7 6 5 4 3 2 1

The paper used in this publication meets minimum requirements of the
American National Standard for Information Sciences—Permanence of Paper
for Printed Library Materials: ANSI Z39.48-1992.

Typeset in Sabon

Composition by Cynthia Stock
Silver Spring, Maryland

Printed by R. R. Donnelley
Harrisonburg, Virginia

Contents

Foreword

Of all the challenges facing the United States, one of the most daunting and important is the growing inadequacy of our national health care system. Sound analysis of the problem and constructive recommendations on the solution—or, as my colleague Hank Aaron would put it, accurate diagnosis combined with effective prescriptions—is a major institutional commitment of the Brookings Institution. We're lucky to have had Hank on our staff since 1967 and on the cutting edge of this issue for the last twenty-six years, and we're proud to be publishing this book as a contribution to the search for better policies in the future.

At the heart of this book's thesis is a paradox. As never before in human history, medical care can enhance the quality and extend the duration of life. It has also become so costly that it can bankrupt governments and impoverish individuals. Until now, Americans have lived under a health care system that told the well insured: if it helps, you deserve it, and someone will pay for it. That roughly 15 percent of the U.S. population is entirely uninsured remains a problem, embarrassment, or scandal, depending on one's point of view. But the complement of that statistic is that 85 percent of the population is insured.

The spate of new medical technology released during the twentieth century promises (or threatens—if one looks at costs) to become a flood in the twenty-first. Now Americans must ask just how much of the benefits of modern medicine they can afford. The challenge is to find ways to ensure that people have access to applications of medical technologies, new and old, that yield benefits greater than cost, while curtailing outlays on health care that costs more than its benefits are worth.

This book offers some clear, cogently argued answers to that question. It compares practices in Great Britain, where health care has long been rationed, with those in the United States, where the idea of denying any well-insured person any beneficial care, however costly, remains explosively controversial. *Can We Say No?* updates and amplifies an earlier study published by Brookings in 1984, *The Painful Prescription: Rationing Hospital Care*, by Hank and William B. Schwartz. While Hank and Melissa Cox wrote the current study, we felt it appropriate to list Bill Schwartz as a coauthor, given his role in the predecessor volume, his participation in some interviews carried out for this one, and his helpful comments on the final manuscript.

Other recent Brookings publications underscore the central role of health care in current and projected budget imbalances. *Restoring Fiscal Sanity: How to Balance the Budget* (2004) and *Restoring Fiscal Sanity: Meeting the Long-Run Challenge* (2005), both edited by Alice Rivlin and Isabel Sawhill, show that federal spending is projected to grow far more than federal revenues and that most of that increase is attributable to anticipated increases in health care spending. Emerging medical technologies and population aging are the principal forces behind these projected increases. Finding ways to slow the growth of public health expenditures without betraying the nation's established commitment to ensure high-quality health care for the aged, disabled, and poor will challenge policymakers for decades to come.

Nor is the challenge of rising health care spending limited to so-called entitlements or even to all government-funded health programs. Per capita private and public health care spending have risen at similar rates. The reason is straightforward. Public and private spending must grow at similar rates if the employed—who are largely covered by private health insurance—and the aged, disabled, and poor—who are covered largely by public programs—are to enjoy roughly comparable care. Avoiding gross discrepancies in the quality of care, based on income, age, or other personal characteristics, has long been a goal of policy in the United States and other developed nations.

Thus, finding ways to curtail low-benefit, high-cost care while ensuring financial access to care for all Americans is a matter of extreme and enduring importance to both the nation's general economic health and to its fiscal stability. So in addition to being part of a long tradition of informing debate on health policy, *Can We Say No?* is also part of our rededication to elevating the attention that the public pays to this issue—and, we hope, contributing to the wisdom of policymakers as they face up to the hard choices facing our nation.

STROBE TALBOTT
President
Brookings Institution

Washington, D.C.
September 2005

Acknowledgments

I owe thanks to many people who have contributed to this volume. Melissa Cox began as a research assistant for this project but became a coauthor thanks to her pervasive contributions based on intimate knowledge of British institutions and sources, as well as her energy, indefatigability, and intelligence.

Alan Garber, Barbara McNeil, Joseph Newhouse, and a fourth referee reviewed the entire manuscript. Howard Glennerster also read the entire manuscript and provided numerous suggestions and corrections, particularly regarding health care arrangements in Great Britain. Dr. Richard Binder also read the entire manuscript and arranged interviews for me and Melissa Cox with colleagues at the INOVA-Fairfax Hospital: Brigit Castro, Alain Drooz, James P. Earls, and Christopher M. Putman. All made numerous remarkably constructive suggestions regarding fact, interpretation, and organization. Particular sections of the book were reviewed by Dr. William Peck, the former dean of the medical school at Washington University in St. Louis, and by his colleagues, Drs. George Broze, John C. Clohisy, Patricia Cole, Daniel Picus, and Marcos Rothstein.

The following physicians from Great Britain, the United States, the Netherlands, and South Africa contributed generously of their time and knowledge through extensive interviews: Andrew Adam, Graeme Bydder, Alexander Davison, Peter Dawson, Adrian Dixon, Simon Eccleshall, John

Feehally, Leon Fine, Howard Freeman, Scott Gazelle, Roger Greenwood, Stewart Higgins, Larry Hollier, Derek Hopper, Janet Husband, James Johnson, Tom Mabin, Rhidian Morris, Andrew Reese, David Hesketh Roberts, Paul Roderick, Christopher White, and Charles van Ypersle. Deborah Zarin with the Agency for Health Research and Quality provided invaluable suggestions and guidance regarding radiology. Karen Garber of the American Hospital Association, Ken Bokina of IMV Medical Information Division, and Mark Brooker of the World Hemophilia Federation each provided specific information and guidance on how to find more. Dr. William Waters participated in some of the interviews.

Gina Russell provided expert research assistance. Kathleen Elliott Yinug scheduled interviews and provided administrative assistance. Starr Belsky edited the manuscript.

The Brookings Institution received funding for this project from the Robert Wood Johnson Foundation's Changes in Health Care Financing and Organization (HFCO) Initiative.

HJA

Can We Say
NO?

CHAPTER ONE

The Promise and the Problem

The good news is that modern medicine works miracles. The bad news is that it breaks banks—public and private. The benefits from improved health care exceed by trillions of dollars its admittedly large and growing cost.[1] Before the late 1960s and the development of durable artificial hips, for example, it was impossible to enable people crippled by painful, arthritic hips to walk normally again. Before the invention of computed tomography (CT) scanners or magnetic resonance imaging (MRI) it was often impossible—short of invasive, painful, and costly exploratory surgery—to pinpoint the exact location of many deep tumors or abscesses. Such procedures generate total costs far higher than the more primitive techniques they replaced but produce enormous gains for many patients. Few Americans would willingly trade today's health care, costly though it is, for the less expensive but less effective treatments of the past.

Still, the cost of these advances is staggering. Real U.S. medical expenditures have increased sevenfold since 1965, when Congress passed Medicare and Medicaid. Outlays will reach $11,046 per person and 18.7 percent of gross domestic product by 2014, according to official projections.[2] If the gap between growth of health care spending and income persists, the former would claim half of all increases in income by 2022 and all of it by 2051. Total health care spending would claim about 28 percent of total U.S. production by 2030 and 35 percent by 2040.[3]

Such rapid growth in spending is not unique—for example, real computer purchases have risen 188-fold since 1978.[4] Although far faster than the increase in health care spending, the increase in computer spending evokes no fretful hand wringing about spiraling computer expenditures. No politician feels driven to orate on the need to contain computer costs. To understand the difference, one need look no further than health insurance. Computer buyers pay directly for each additional machine they buy. Health care consumers do not: on average, patients pay out-of-pocket for only 3 percent of hospital care and 11 percent of physician services.[5] And during serious illnesses, when out-of-pocket spending exceeds defined limits, many insurance plans now pay all costs of care. To be sure, when health costs rise, the cost of health insurance—private and public—goes up. But the prospect of such charges has little influence on the amount of care that well-insured patients seek when ill or that their caregivers are disposed to render.

Insurance protects people from financial ruination by health care costs. Indeed, it is the lack of such coverage by some 45 million people that troubles elected officials and everyone else, even if agreement on how to extend coverage has proven elusive. In addition to—indeed, precisely because of—such financial protection, insurance produces two side effects. First, by shielding patients from all or most of the cost of care, insurance encourages patients to demand all care, however small the benefit and however high the cost of producing it. Sometimes such care—the test that provides additional information of little value, the medicine that is trivially better than a much less costly alternative, the surgery that is expected to produce only small improvements—generates benefits that are, in some sense, smaller than the costs.[6] And as medical technology improves and total benefits from advancing technology increase, outlays on care that does not deliver value for money also will tend to increase. Second, health insurance also relieves biomedical investigators of any need to worry about the cost of new and better treatments.

Victor Fuchs and Alan Garber vividly illustrate the working of these two unintended side effects of insurance:

> Imagine how the market for automobiles would have developed if a third party had provided automobile insurance that paid 80 percent of the cost of new cars. . . . Such insurance would influence both the number and types of cars people bought. People would replace cars more often, and they would buy higher quality cars

than they do in today's automobile market. A Lincoln or a Mercedes would cost buyers little more than a Chevrolet or a Honda, and sales of luxury automobiles would rise. Auto manufacturers would focus their product development on quality enhancements, such as big engines and luxurious interiors, rather than on cost-reducing manufacturing changes. . . . The quality-adjusted price of automobiles might fall, but since only high-quality cars would be sold, the average price of a car would rise. . . . The well-insured might welcome the steady improvements in the quality of luxury cars, but many would be better off with simpler automobiles and higher take-home pay.[7]

The enormous benefits and costs of prospective medical advances magnify the importance of reaching three goals. The first is to ensure that all Americans enjoy financial access to modern health care. That means extending health insurance to the currently uninsured and upgrading coverage for those who now are inadequately insured. Achieving this goal will doubtless add to health care spending. The second goal is to ensure that all patients receive care that is worth what it costs. The failure of the U.S. health care system to meet this standard, even for the well insured, is increasingly well documented. The third goal is to eliminate care that is not worth what it costs.

Achievement of universal coverage is likely to be a necessary precursor to eliminating care that is not worth what it costs. The uninsured now receive substantial amounts of free or subsidized care that is financed by extra charges levied on the insured. Such cross-subsidies provide the modicum of protection for the uninsured without which the status of being uninsured would be intolerable. Yet aggressive efforts to control costs for the insured inevitably constrict the capacity of health care providers to sustain such "unreimbursed" care. Effective cost control would also require control mechanisms that do not currently exist in the United States.

The practical questions concern how to curtail such care. Public policy could limit demand for care—for example, by withdrawing tax concessions that lower the cost of health insurance or by raising the price of care through higher premiums or increased charges at the time of use. The legislation enacted in 2003 to encourage high-deductible insurance is an example of such an approach. However, demand restriction suffers from a serious shortcoming. Any insurance that effectively protects people from financial catastrophe must pay for essentially all costs beyond a limit. Most health costs are incurred by a small proportion of the population whose expenses greatly exceed plausible limits on out-of-pocket spending. Demand-limiting strategies can deter spending up to a point but can exercise no influence at the margin on care provided once costs exceed such limits. For that reason, demand limitations are likely to have only a modest impact on the development and deployment of new medical technologies.

The second general approach, to curb the advance of medical technology—for example, by curtailing public support of basic science—would be neither desirable nor effective. It is not desirable because, as noted, the average benefits of advancing medical technology are likely in the future, as they have been in the past, to greatly exceed their costs. It is not likely to be effective because the United States is not the only sponsor of medical research. Other nations would be ready and are increasingly able to entice top investigators with research support if the United States cuts off such funding. Therefore, curtailing biomedical research in the United States would sacrifice scientific leadership without achieving the intended reduction in cost-increasing health technology.

The third approach to controlling growth in health care spending is to try to limit the provision of care that is worth less than it costs people who are well insured—that is, to ration care. Other nations commonly use budgetary limits or restrict the supply of key personnel or equipment so that health care providers must limit care. The current maze of ways Americans pay for health care is incapable of enforcing such limits. To create such controls would precipitate passionate debate centered on deep ideological divisions over the proper scope for collective authority and individual rights.

Thus the steps necessary to ration health care may prove more objectionable than the cost of paying for it. But as the health care menu lengthens, the cost of low-benefit care that well-insured patients will demand under current payment arrangements is likely to become so burdensome that serious examination of health care rationing and what it would take to implement it will prove inescapable. The outcome of such a debate cannot be prejudged. But to discuss the options intelligently, Americans need to understand not just the size of the economic challenge but also the choices that health care rationing will entail. This book is an attempt to provide readers with such information.

Some History

Rapid growth of health care expenditures has led successive presidents to propose limits on hospital outlays or other medical spending. The administrations of presidents Nixon, Ford, Carter, Reagan, and Clinton proposed to limit growth of health care spending through a number of means: price controls (Nixon), hospital revenue controls (Nixon and Carter), limits on Medicare and Medicaid spending, and increased competition (Reagan and George W. Bush), or sweeping reform (Clinton). On a parallel track, Congress tried to slow growth of medical expenditures by requiring states to discourage duplication of medical facilities by having care providers obtain a certificate of need from the local health system agencies before making a capital expenditure greater than $100,000 or $150,000. State governments introduced mandatory controls on hospital charges, third-party payment rates, or total hospital revenue. The state programs all proved unsustainable and lapsed or languished because none succeeded in limiting outlays more than briefly.

The two most enduring efforts to control costs have been Medicare's shift from cost-based reimbursement to prospective payment systems and private sector adoption of managed care. Until 1983 Medicare paid hospitals based on costs incurred. In that year it began to pay hospitals fixed amounts set prospectively for most in-patient services and based on patients' diagnoses at time of admission. These fees have been adjusted annually based on changes in the cost of hospitals' inputs, hospital productivity, and other considerations. Initial prices were quite generous, but Medicare gradually used this system to slow spending growth. Medicare later established fee schedules for physician services. Still later it extended prospective payment to hospital outpatient services, home health providers, and skilled nursing facilities.[8]

The second cost control effort played out in the private sector. In the 1990s private payers began to try to control costs through private regulatory devices grouped under the term *managed care*. This term includes the cost control methods of health maintenance organizations that provide all or most care through salaried or contractual staff. It encompasses preferred provider organizations that encourage enrollees to use designated providers who offer discounts. It also covers the efforts by insurers or plan managers to limit fees, screen patients for particular services, and negotiate discounts from suppliers, physicians, and other health professionals. At about the time that these practices became wide-spread, growth of health care spending decelerated. Whether this slow-down resulted from or simply coincided with managed care is unclear. That the slowdown was short lived is not. People objected to the aggres-sive cost control methods used by managed care companies. Personal tes-timonies, news reports, and movies made managed care an object of fear and loathing for many people who objected to the denial of care by busi-ness executives and even physicians who stood to gain financially from their parsimony. The plans scaled back efforts to control costs.

Rapid growth of per capita health care spending—which has outpaced income growth by an average of 2.5 percent annually since 1960—resumed in 2000. This excess growth seems likely to persist until and unless the U.S. public is prepared to tolerate effective cost limits, private or public. To be sure, spending growth has slowed episodically in the past and may do so in the future. The reduction of wasteful practices could achieve sizable, but one-time, savings. A slowdown in the advance of medical technology and the attendant flow of new therapeutic and diag-nostic procedures would also slow the growth of health care spending. But such a slowdown seems highly improbable in light of the recent breakthroughs in molecular and cellular biology and in information tech-nology. More importantly, it would be a misfortune because it would mean that humans were deprived of the life-extending, pain-reducing, and function-enhancing contributions that have defined medical advance.

Rationing

What this all means is that a *sustained* slowdown in the growth of health care spending will require rationing—the denial of some beneficial care to some people who have the financial means to pay for it. Such rationing should not be confused with the absence of health insurance for millions of Americans. Many observers characterize this situation as "rationing by price." But the term *rationing* ordinarily does not refer to the inability of some people in a market economy to afford particular commodities. Cus-tomarily, it describes the situation in which people who can afford a com-modity are unable to buy it because of scarcity, which results because some nonmarket allocation system—ration coupons or queues, for exam-ple—limits demand to available supply.

No other nation spends nearly as much on health care as does the United States. Per capita health care spending in the United States, at

$5,267 in 2002, was more than twice the $2,049 average of other members of the Organization for Economic Cooperation and Development (OECD) and more than half again as great as spending in the second highest spending nation—Switzerland ($3,446).[9] These differentials are attributable to several causes. First, U.S. physicians receive particularly generous remuneration. Second, rich nations may spend a larger share of their incomes on health care than do poorer nations, and the United States is richer than most other OECD nations.[10] Third, the United States tends to have more medical equipment and higher rates of surgery than do most other nations.

Other wealthy nations limit health care spending in various ways. The highly decentralized U.S. payment system is unique in its lack of effective levers for limiting health care spending. The theme of this book is that the United States will be forced by sharply rising public and private health care spending to consider the adoption of such limits. Even if the total benefits from advancing medical technology far outweigh the total costs, the amount spent on care that provides only marginal benefits is likely to grow even faster (see chapter 6). For this reason, the stakes in controlling health care spending will increase even as the benefits from advancing medical technology grow. Limits, whatever their particular form, will require that some sick people be denied some care that is somewhat beneficial but worth less than it costs.

To understand whether the rationing "cure" is less painful than the "disease" of sharply higher taxes and private health care spending, one must understand what sorts of trade-offs rationing requires. U.S. experience offers scant guidance because the well-insured now enjoy financial access to essentially all beneficial care. Nor do the uninsured offer a good indication of what rationing would entail, as whatever care they receive comes from hospitals and physicians whose practice patterns are shaped by the financial incentives resulting from the majority, who are well insured.

To secure insight on the implications of health care rationing, one must look at a system in which resources are limited for all. The British health care system provides such a perspective. The United States is unlikely to adopt the particular institutional arrangements that the British have used to control health care spending or to ration care as severely. Other developed nations employ different methods for controlling spending, and few have rationed care as stringently as have the British. For that reason, the British experience provides a clearer view of the kinds of trade-offs that rationing entails. The final chapter describes various ways in which rationing might be implemented in the United States and the results likely in the U.S. context. Before then, however, it is essential to see what rationing would entail.

Lessons from Britain

Important similarities between Britain and the United States suggest that British reactions to resource limits will provide some guidance to probable U.S. reactions to such limits. Each country's medical journals are commonly read in the other. The clinical and scientific standards of both nations are similar. Some physicians from each country spend time in the other as students, teachers, and researchers.

Despite these similarities, British and American societies are not identical. Britain has rigidly controlled medical expenditures for decades.[11] Per capita hospital expenditures are now about 45 percent of those in the United States.[12] For decades such limits have shaped British medical practice and patient attitudes, forcing the British to decide what medical services *not* to provide, a challenge that the United States so far has declined to confront. The organization of health care, the political system, and the relative importance of class differ between the two nations. British patients are less demanding of their health care providers and less litigious than Americans, although these dissimilarities may be narrowing. For these reasons, British behavior is not an exact model for the choices Americans would make if the United States sought to severely curb medical expenditures.

Chapter 2 describes the British health care system for American readers. To measure the practical results of budget limits, chapters 3 through 5 compare the provision of representative health procedures in the United States and Britain.[13] This book is based on the assumption that U.S. service levels provide a benchmark for treatment levels if well-insured patients receive all care expected to generate net medical benefits. To be sure, Medicare's prospective payment system, private managed care, and capitated health plans can discourage the provision of some beneficial care. Medicare's prospective payment system means that hospitals do not receive larger payments if they provide additional services (other than extra payments for unusually costly cases). Some health care organizations use financial incentives to discourage what they regard as excessive care. Others require prior approval for some treatments as a condition for payment. But the large majority of Americans receive care under plans that have few tools to control spending. The system of cost-based reimbursement encourages the provision to most patients of all care that promises to yield benefits, regardless of cost.

In some instances, the U.S. system provides more than all beneficial care. Huge geographic variations in the provision of many forms of health care persist that differences in rates of illness cannot explain. Studies indicate that outcomes in regions of particularly heavy use are no better than elsewhere.[14] Such evidence strongly suggests that too much care is provided in some places. The fear of being sued may cause some physicians to practice defensive medicine, that is, to provide care designed more to minimize the risk of being sued than to improve patient outcomes. Other physicians may perform surgery they consider of marginal value or recommend unnecessary tests in order to boost their own incomes. The extent or even existence of these practices remains a matter of controversy.[15] On balance, however, care in the United States for most well-insured patients still remains close to what would be provided if cost were no object and benefit to patients were the sole concern.

Given this assumption, the British system is deemed to provide "full care" if its service levels are similar to those in the United States. The difference is a measure of rationing. The practical question is whether those differences make medical and social sense. Chapter 6 lays out an analytical framework for thinking about these questions and presents estimates of the degree to which differences in the provision of the procedures examined in chapters 3 through 5 account for the large difference between U.S. and British health care expenditures.

What to Look For

Chapters 3, 4, and 5 reveal gaps of widely varying sizes between the United States and Britain in the availability of several medical services. These chapters also explore possible medical justifications or other explanations for these differences. The data are inadequate to test in a statistically rigorous way precisely why the British limit various forms of care to such different degrees. Readers should decide whether the reasons presented here are plausible. They should also decide whether they think that people in the United States would respond similarly or differently.

Some observed behaviors are ones that any budget-limited system would elicit. Physicians who say "no" must learn to do so in ways that are acceptable both to themselves and to their patients. Patients unwilling to accept the consequences of resource limits are likely to seek ways to "work the system" to secure care they were initially denied. Communities may circumvent limits by donating equipment that would not otherwise be available. Interest groups may use the media to try to pressure the government to increase allocations for the treatment of certain diseases. Chapter 7 summarizes British responses to limits on health care, while chapter 8 considers how such responses would affect the operation of budget limits in the United States.

Chapters 7 and 8 also address several other complex questions. Should patients be permitted to buy medical care outside a system subject to budget limits? Can clinical freedom survive in an environment of budget limits? Should charitable gifts always be welcomed? What legal actions would arise because of effective budget limits? How should limits be structured so that physicians and patients operate within them, rather than working to defeat them?

Control of health care spending involves many technical issues. For example, hospital spending can be controlled with fixed budgets, revenue limits per patient day, or revenue limits per admission. Alternatively, demand for hospitalization can be influenced by deductibles and co-payments of various kinds. Each control mechanism creates particular incentives and distortions. The choice among them is of fundamental importance. This volume does not deal with such issues. The focus, rather, is on those decisions and trade-offs that must be made if budget limits are to be effective. Primary emphases are on behavioral adjustments that must be encouraged, institutional changes that would result, the value judgments that budget limits would require, and the coping mechanisms that they would elicit. How far the United States will—or should—venture in rationing medical care is unclear. That it will have to confront this difficult problem is beyond dispute.

CHAPTER TWO

The British System

In a famous exchange, Ernest Hemingway wryly responded to F. Scott Fitzgerald's observation that "the rich are different from you and me" by saying, "Yes, they have more money." In comparing the American and British health care systems, a Fitzgerald-like comment would be that the health systems of the two nations differ because of history, politics, and medical institutions. A Hemingway-like response would be that Americans spend more than twice as much as the British do.[1]

Although Britain spends far less per capita on medical care than does the United States, it has 13 percent more acute care hospital beds per capita, 64 percent as many doctors, 55 percent as many nurses, 25 percent more admissions to acute care hospitals, and similar length hospital stays.[2] Crude indicators of health status put Britain abreast or slightly ahead of the United States. Life expectancy at birth was higher and infant mortality was lower in Great Britain than in the United States in the year 2000.[3]

Such measures do not necessarily mean that the British health care system is better or worse than that in the United States—just different. Clearly, however, money alone does not buy longevity. Health depends more on income and nutrition, genetics, personal habits, and the environment than on what doctors and hospitals do.[4]

Formation of the National Health Service

The National Health Service was created in the wake of the devastation and privation of World War II, a socially and politically seminal event, as well as an economic and military trauma, that profoundly changed British political and social attitudes toward health care and much else. For the first time in their lives, wounded soldiers and civilians were granted free, high-quality medical care. Even at the start of the war, surveys indicated a national consensus that ensuring access to health care was a government responsibility. The Beveridge Report of 1942, which advocated free and universal health services, was used both to boost morale at home and to tantalize the enemy with visions of a superior British system. More generally, military victory, which succeeded two decades of economic stagnation (the specifically British slump of the 1920s and the worldwide depression of the 1930s) was widely regarded as a triumph of state planning.

The public regarded governmental provision of health care as natural and fair, and the successful prosecution of the war made it seem that government could do the job.[5] The Labour Party, running on a platform calling for state ownership of basic industries, won a staggering political victory in the first postwar election. A leading plank in the Labour platform was the promised National Health Service.

For these reasons, the creation of the National Health Service (NHS) in 1948 provoked strikingly little controversy. A major exception was the opposition of the British Medical Association, whose spokesmen warned that government control would interfere with physician autonomy. But the Royal Colleges, representing the various medical specialties, overcame this resistance, perhaps because health minister Aneurin Bevan agreed to permit admission of private patients to NHS hospitals and to allow part-time private practice, a particular boon to specialists. The public solidly supported government management of health. In fact, more than 80 percent of the British public had endorsed a national health system in 1941, well before the Beveridge Plan enunciated the idea as a national goal. As early as 1911, then–prime minister Lloyd George had introduced a plan that provided national coverage of general practitioner services for workers but excluded spouses and children.[6]

Seven lean years followed the creation of the NHS, during which the British economy struggled to recover from wartime destruction and dislocations. The share of income devoted to health fell slowly. Then ensued two robust, if not fat, decades lasting into the 1970s. Public health spending rose from 3.6 percent of gross domestic product in 1954 to 5.6 percent in 1980. From then until the end of the century, outlays rose somewhat faster than gross domestic product, reaching 7.6 percent of GDP in 2001.[7] Although British health care spending grew faster than in other countries, such as France and Germany, it started from a much lower base and remained lower than in all other northern European nations. Meanwhile, outlays in the United States tripled as a share of GDP between 1960 and 2003, going from 5.1 to 15.3 percent.[8] Adjusted for age, the gap between British and U.S. spending was even larger than these numbers suggest because the elderly form a larger share of the British than U.S. population.[9]

In evaluating the NHS, British citizens could look to the past or they could look abroad. Immediately after the war, the British tended to compare availability of care with what they had before, not with the standards of other countries. The NHS was an egalitarian oasis in a class-ridden society, promising high-quality medical care to the acutely ill, regardless of class. It delivered on that promise and shielded the sick and dying from financial ruin by medical bills. The NHS also oversaw a steady improvement in health care quality, even if constrained British health budgets limited access to the trove of new technology that became available in the late twentieth century. In the words of historian Geoffrey Rivett,

> We take the National Health Service for granted now, but it is only a little over fifty years ago that health care was a luxury not everyone could afford. It is difficult today for us to imagine what life must have been like without free health care and the difference that the arrival of the NHS made to people's lives. . . . Poor people who previously often went without medical treatment, relying instead on dubious and sometimes dangerous home remedies or on the charity of doctors who gave their services free to their poorest patients, now had access to services.[10]

The number of admissions doubled between 1949 and 1967. The fruits of medical research transformed the character of medical care.[11] Wealthy foreigners, who understood that some of the world's best health services could be found in Britain, came to seek treatment. For these achievements, the NHS became and remained one of the most popular institutions in Britain, second only to the Crown—and a close second at that.[12]

Spending grew, but less rapidly than the cost of providing all sick people with the benefits of all new medical procedures. For most routine contacts with the health system—visits to general practitioners and clear emergencies—the majority of the British had better access to care than ever before and better than did the millions of uninsured Americans. But many with chronic or nonemergency conditions, even quite painful or debilitating ones, languished on growing waiting lists. Class differences in the use of health care continued, despite removal of financial barriers to access. Geographic variation in the availability of care remained almost as large a quarter century after the creation of the NHS as it had been at its inception. The typical British hospital around 1980 was Edwardian or older. The relative remuneration of physicians was falling. Starting in 1975, fiscal duress forced successive governments, both Labour and Conservative, to curtail growth of health care spending. Discontent intensified as queues lengthened and awareness spread that the gap between British spending and that in other countries was not closing.

Then, starting in 1976, successive governments instituted a series of major changes. The first came with the shift in funding among health regions recommended by the Resource Allocation Working Party (RAWP). RAWP sought to reduce disparities in health outcomes among regions by shifting funds to those with relatively poor outcomes. Reductions in geographic disparities within regions remained beyond reach because adequate data to deal with them were lacking and because class inequities remained too controversial to touch. Nonetheless, the RAWP formula signaled a break with the tradition-driven allocation of funds that had prevailed for the preceding three decades.

In the late 1980s, the Conservative government of Prime Minister Margaret Thatcher instituted major administrative changes. The Thatcher government did not accelerate spending growth or change the principle of need-based geographic allocations financed from central taxation. Instead, it introduced elements of market-type competition into the management of the National Health Service. These changes, it was claimed, would expand and improve health care for any given outlay. The study of whether the Thatcher reforms had their intended effect became a cottage industry for academics. The net verdict of numerous studies is mixed: costs may have been reduced, but quality may have suffered.[13]

When the Labour party returned to office in 1997, it preserved a key Thatcher innovation—the separation between purchase and provision of health care—but modified another—the designation of the general practitioner as the financial manager for most health care. If Britain could not "reform its way" to better health care, the inescapable conclusion was that more money would be necessary to modernize the system. That is just what the Blair government started to do in 2000. One-third of health service buildings dated from before the creation of the NHS in 1948. To modernize facilities, the Blair government undertook what it characterized as the largest hospital building program in the history of the NHS.[14] It set in place a plan to increase real health care spending by an average of 6.1 percent annually through 2004, later revised upward to 7.2 percent for the five fiscal years ending in 2007–08.[15] It promised to bring the U.K. share of GDP devoted to health care up to the anticipated unweighted average among European members of the Organization for Economic Cooperation and Development by 2004 and to continue rapid increases thereafter.[16]

How the National Health Service Works

Every developed industrial country has fashioned arrangements that protect all of its population against the full costs of health care at the time of illness—the exception being the United States, where most, but not all of the population has some kind of protection. Along with its benefits, insurance creates related problems.

The first is the need to find some way to limit spending on medical care. This problem arises because fully insured patients have no reason when ill to concern themselves about costs—someone else pays for their care. Even if insurance is incomplete, it spares seriously ill patients from most or all of what it costs to produce medical care. Patients who act like normal consumers will seek care as long as their benefits exceed what they pay. They have little cause to attend to the much larger cost of producing the services they use. Accordingly, insured patients are likely to use some care that costs more to produce than it is worth to them. But preventing such waste requires some form of external control, and such controls are also costly. All well-insured nations must choose how much to tolerate waste that arises when care is free or nearly free at time of use and how much to spend to avoid such waste.[17]

The second problem is how to ensure that health care is produced efficiently. Efficiency has multiple dimensions. It means that providers select the particular services that achieve given health outcomes at the lowest feasible cost. It means that those services are produced with the fewest possible resources. (The concept of efficiency is described in more detail in chapter 6).

A third issue—the desirability of equality—has been particularly salient in Great Britain and has shaped debates over organization of the National Health Service.[18] Whether equality refers to per capita spending, spending adjusted for illness, or health outcomes has rarely been clear. Yet clarity on this matter is critical because the implications of these standards are quite dissimilar. Indeed, equality of health outcomes, given enormous genetic and environmental diversity, is probably impossible and would certainly result in poorer overall health outcomes than if some inequality were tolerated. But one of the enduring appeals of the National Health Service is that it rests on a shared objective of ensuring access to care that is more equal and fair than the system it replaced or than alternatives in other nations, notably the United States.

Finances

The National Health Service is mostly supported by government funds: 74 percent from general revenues; 20 percent from earmarked involuntary contributions by individuals and their employers on behalf of each person covered under the NHS; 2 percent from charges imposed for dentistry, drugs, and a few other items; and 4 percent from other sources.[19] Because much of the population—including children, the elderly and disabled, and people on low incomes—is exempt from NHS drug charges, 85 percent of prescriptions are dispensed for free.[20]

Until the Thatcher reforms, the government financed and administered the National Health Service through three distinct government channels. General practitioners (GPs) received a flat per patient fee that covered the cost of primary care only. They typically practiced in small groups. Each patient signed up with a particular GP practice, which provided all primary care at no charge to the patient. Patients could not go to other GPs unless they formally switched. Nor could they go to specialists for free services unless referred by their GPs. A small proportion of specialists saw patients privately for a fee that patients had to pay themselves. The NHS paid separately for drugs, which all physicians could prescribe.

Hospital and other institutional care was separately funded. In England such care was financed by governmental appropriations funneled through fourteen regions and thence through 192 districts. Hospital budgets accounted for two-thirds of NHS expenditures. Hospitals employed all specialists on a salaried basis. They carried out essentially all tests requiring advanced equipment. The quantity of such tests was therefore determined by the level of hospital budgets. Finally, nonhospital community care was provided by district nurses and health visitors, financed and administered by local authorities.

Budget Setting: Old Style

From its inception, NHS spending was set by Parliament for the entire United Kingdom. Parliament determined NHS budgets until 1999 when it devolved these powers to the Scottish Parliament and the National Assembly for Wales. Until the Thatcher reforms, expenditures of each hospital were also largely determined by national budgets that were funneled to health regions and districts. These budgets could be supplemented from three other sources: charity; "pay beds," that is, revenues from private payers who used some beds in NHS facilities; and, in the case of some teaching hospitals, endowments, mostly acquired before the creation of the NHS.

The overall NHS budget emerges from a multiyear plan influenced strongly by spending levels in previous years. The British Treasury, which combines functions of the U.S. Department of the Treasury and the Office of Management and Budget, determines whether the NHS budget and that of other government agencies should increase and, if so, how much. The cabinet modifies and approves the full budget, which is then submitted to the House of Commons. The final budget differs little from the government's proposal for two reasons. First, the budget of the Chancellor of the Exchequer cannot be amended on the floor. Second, party discipline is applied to budget votes. The budget is divided into two parts, one for new construction and capital equipment and one for current operations. Authority to move funds between these categories is strictly limited. The resulting health appropriation is a global budget for the National Health Service.

In the pre-Thatcher days, most funds were transferred successively from the Treasury to subsidiary geographically based units, the number and organization of which changed periodically. Decisions about hospital equipment or services that covered more than one district, such as blood banks, computed tomography scanners, or coronary artery surgery, were determined nationally or regionally. Increases in hospital medical staff required regional approval, which was hard to get because authorities believed that limiting hospital staffs was the best way to control the budget. Each jurisdiction had to absorb the higher costs from unanticipated inflation. Districts or regions that overspent their budgets were docked the next period. A second adjustment accounted for movement of patients across jurisdictional boundaries: each region was reimbursed an amount equal to its net "imports" multiplied by the average cost of patient care.

Under this system, each hospital's budget typically equaled that of the preceding year, plus an inflation and population adjustment, unless it could make a strong case for an addition. Hospital administrators and staff had to "eat" the costs of unanticipated inflation by deferring maintenance (painting cycles, for example, sometimes stretched to decades), delaying replacement of equipment, or leaving staff positions unfilled. Large expenditures—new hospitals, for example—or expenditures on experimental procedures were likely to be made at a higher jurisdiction, such as the region.

Because real national health care spending grew slowly, a budget increase for one facility came at the expense of another. Creative local health officials could add marginally to their own resources without reducing someone else's only by stimulating charitable contributions. By and large, however, budget limits were binding.

The traditional way in which hospitals and districts were run also furthered the achievement of budget targets. British hospitals were quasi-feudal enterprises, ruled largely by a peerage of senior specialist physicians, called "consultants." Most spent their careers at one hospital and derived all of their income from salary. Most had junior physicians assigned to them and controlled a certain number of beds to which they alone could admit patients. Directly or indirectly, they controlled almost all the hospital's resources. Typical British hospital administrators, unlike their U.S. counterparts, lacked power or authority. Thus consultants, whose personal salaries and positions were little affected by budgetary vicissitudes, parceled out the meager rations allotted through the health district. They had every incentive to do so amicably, for they belonged to a select medical club whose members had to work together, usually for the rest of their professional lives. That each had only a limited personal economic stake in the outcome of the allocations facilitated such cooperation.

A minority of consultants, mostly in the southwest and mostly in a few specialties, such as surgery, supplemented their incomes from private practices. Stringent NHS budgets that resulted in long queues for some services could be manipulated to drive patients to the private sector and increase consultants' incomes from private practice.

Budget Setting: New Style

The reforms initiated under Prime Minister Thatcher and continued in modified form by Prime Minister Tony Blair have introduced a measure of flexibility into what was an extremely rigid process. Separate parliaments for England and Scotland continue to legislate annual budgets that limit NHS spending. Patients still must sign up with a particular general practitioner who acts as gatekeeper for specialist care. Under the Thatcher system, GPs were still paid on a capitation basis, based on the number of enrollees, but GP groups were given greatly increased financial responsibility as so-called fundholders—essentially group practices that received increased capitation payments to cover not only primary care but also prescriptions and nonemergency hospital care. Not all GPs accepted this financial responsibility, but those who did became physician case managers responsible for handling the costs not only of primary care but also for elective procedures and outpatient drugs. GPs could choose among hospitals for their patients.[21]

The successor Labour government in 1997 ended the devolution of part of hospital budgets to GP fundholding groups. The government instead created new Primary Care Trusts (PCTs) in England. These new organizations were essentially health authorities, in many cases serving areas smaller than the districts they replaced. The PCTs are responsible for most of the health services for populations and dispose of approximately three quarters of NHS spending in each area. They fund not just hospital and community services but also drugs and primary care. They sign contracts with NHS hospitals to provide a certain quantity of care at a set budget. PCTs with older and more deprived populations receive extra funding because needy populations make disproportionate use of free services.

On paper, PCTs had power to influence hospitals by shifting their business from one competitor to another. But few did so, in part because the government did not encourage such strategies, in part because few hospitals had enough excess capacity to accommodate new clients. The Labour government relied instead on centrally defined performance targets—such as reduction in waiting times—to motivate managers and consultants to improve quality of care.

After trying this approach for a few years, the government reintroduced measures to increase competition among NHS hospitals. Private providers were offered contracts to clear NHS waiting lists. Most significantly, patients were to be offered a choice of hospital, including private ones, for a range of treatments. The hospital was to be paid a fee for services rendered. The fee was to be set in a manner similar to the U.S. system of diagnosis related groups, based on severity of condition. Plans were to try the system first in London and then extend it nationally, starting in 2005. Consultants remain firmly in control of hospital operations, but increased patient choice and sharper competition may erode this. Hospitals are becoming "foundation trusts," empowered to borrow directly from the capital markets up to set limits and to sell off assets, using the proceeds as the hospital wishes.

The Patient

Each English resident enrolls with one of approximately 35,000 GPs.[22] Patients may choose any doctor who has an opening. They may switch when they wish, but few do so. A visit to a GP has normally been the first point of contact with the health care system during any spell of illness. GPs carried an average of 1,666 patients in 2004.[23] GPs may prescribe medications or send specimens to hospital laboratories for analysis. In most cases, however, they cannot order complicated tests or admit patients to a hospital.

If GPs find indications of illness that require more extensive testing or treatment than they can provide from their offices, they refer the patient to a consultant—a specialist, in American parlance. Nearly all specialists who see patients through the NHS are employed by hospital trusts on a salaried basis. GPs may write a letter to consultants or telephone them. If the case is urgent, patients are seen immediately. Otherwise, waits to see consultants have been lengthy—up to five months or even more.[24] To avoid the usual waits, patients may go directly to hospital emergency rooms. After examination, a consultant may prescribe further outpatient tests or treatments, schedule admission to the hospital, or admit a patient immediately.

Waiting Lists

Waiting lists have been perhaps the most notorious aspect of the National Health Service since its inception. By 1950 more than half a million people were waiting for admission to NHS hospitals.[25] In 1999 more than 1.2 million people were awaiting inpatient or day case treatment in England, and waiting lists and times tended to be worse in Ireland, Wales, and Scotland.[26] The number of people on this and other waiting lists is less informative than are the average, median, and maximum times spent on such lists. British waiting list statistics shock Americans but have been improving and, in some respects, are exemplary. Three quarters of ambulance calls are responded to within eight minutes, and more than 96 percent of patients are seen within four hours after an accident or in an emergency. But the number of people awaiting specialist and hospital care and the time they have to wait remain problematic, not least to the British government, which is struggling to improve the situation.

Currently, the NHS collects data on waiting lists or times to see primary care physicians and specialists, to receive outpatient or day care from hospitals, and to be admitted for inpatient care. The outpatient waiting list includes people whom GPs have referred to consultants but who have not yet had their first consultant appointment. The inpatient waiting list includes patients whom consultants have decided need to be admitted to a hospital but who have not yet been admitted.[27] Other waits—for diagnostic tests, for example—are not officially measured and are referred to as "hidden waits."

The number of people on each list has fluctuated widely, as has the duration of stays on each list. The number of people on the outpatient waiting list for at least three months reached a maximum of more than half a million. By 2003 that number had been cut more than two-thirds. In 1999 more than 150,000 people were on the outpatient list for more than six months. By 2003 waits of that duration were substantially eliminated.

Progress on the inpatient list is clear, but the situation is still troubling. Between the early 1980s and 1998, the inpatient waiting list swelled from almost 700,000 to more than 1.2 million. After repeated initiatives, the Blair administration has reduced the inpatient list below 1 million, although nearly 20 percent were on the waiting list for more than six months. Some of the reduction in the total on the list may be an artifact of changed reporting procedures.[28] On the other hand, considerable progress has been made in reducing waiting time for treatment of cancer and selected other diseases. All hospitals claim that they treat children with cancer within one month, as well as those adults whose physicians refer them "urgently."[29]

Some have argued that waiting list data overstate the number of people waiting for hospital admission. Lists often include patients who have deferred admission for medical reasons, have medical problems that may be resolved without hospital admission (such as infertility), have moved away, and, in some instances, have already had treatment.[30] Even patients who die or whose conditions have improved may remain on waiting lists. The names of the chronically ill whose regular and scheduled treatment is set for a later date may also appear on waiting lists.

Given these qualifications, waiting list statistics still portray a problem that remains serious despite significant improvements in the past several years. The number of people on lists may mean little more than that the number of patients served has increased, as all nonemergency patients spend some time on waiting lists. Although waiting times remain problematic, they are decreasing: waits of extreme duration, especially for cancer and a few other diseases, are less frequent now than in the past. The Blair government promised to eliminate waits of more than six months for inpatient care and waits of more than three months for outpatient consultation by the end of 2005, and waits of more than three months for both inpatient and day care by 2008. That the progress in meeting such targets led the King's Fund to the verdict of "greater progress on reducing waiting times than at any other stage in NHS history" testifies to the seriousness of the problem that existed.[31]

Regional Inequalities

For many years, British health planners tried to equalize expenditures among the regions. More recently, they have tried to equalize health. This goal requires large shifts of outlays to areas that are poorer or sicker than average.

At the inception of the NHS, some parts of Britain had new or endowed hospitals and an ample supply of physicians. Other areas were much less fortunate. To improve the distribution of physicians, the NHS provided bonuses for general practitioners who set up practice in underserved areas. Yet this step did little to narrow the regional inequality of hospital expenditures. In the mid-1970s, the difference in per capita hospital spending was nearly as great as when the NHS began.[32] In fact, evaluation of medical services based on NHS spending alone may understate geographic variations because regions with above-average spending also have most of the endowed voluntary hospitals that appear to have been disproportionate beneficiaries of charitable gifts.

In 1976 the specially appointed Resource Allocation Working Party recommended gradual elimination of regional differences in per capita expenditures, adjusted for medical need based on age-specific mortality rates. The government of Prime Minister Thatcher reduced the weight given to mortality rates and introduced a new factor that called for higher payments to regions with high wages or living costs, a shift that worked to the benefit of the already relatively well-endowed London region. Few fundamental changes were made in the formula for allocating funds until the 1990s, when the allocation formula was refined to equalize spending within smaller geographic units.

The Blair government shifted policy fundamentally from one of equalizing access to health care to one of seeking to equalize health. Although equalization policy has shifted, statistics tell an unambiguous story. First, actual fund allocations increasingly matched targets.[33] Second, the focus of funds on the poor did not increase.[34] Third, gaps in mortality rates among social classes and even among geographic areas have widened somewhat in the last three decades.[35]

Summary

British patients and physicians have been, and remain, participants in a structured social and medical care system. Patients ordinarily lack direct access to specialists through the NHS. They normally must first see general practitioners, a custom that predates the NHS. Patients retain the option to see specialists outside the NHS if they are prepared to pay for services themselves, but sequential referral remains a powerful instrument of cost control.

That system is undergoing profound change. Once bound by custom and by a long-term dependency on their GPs, British patients, who were conditioned to accept the authority of family physicians and prestigious consultants, are becoming more insistent in their personal demands. Like Americans, British patients increasingly use hospital emergency rooms to secure primary care.

By contrast, U.S. patients may ordinarily see any doctor with whom they can get an appointment, although some managed care plans employ primary care physicians or nurses as gatekeepers. Many specialists also provide primary care, such as routine checkups and examinations. In contrast to the British, American patients are likely to "doctor shop," seeking out different doctors for different problems. They seem to regard doctors as technicians who are periodically called on to repair their physical machinery, to be dropped if they are unable to solve the current problem or be sued if they botched the last one.

A generation ago, British physicians, many of whom have studied or practiced in the United States, repeatedly said that British patients were more likely than their American counterparts to accept a doctor's judgment as final. British physicians now report that younger patients are becoming more demanding. Perhaps individualism or a New World "Prometheanism"—an unwillingness to acknowledge that there may be no effective human intervention for certain illnesses—is spreading internationally.[36] Regardless, attitudinal differences survive—and so do restraints on patient access to specialists. These differences not only embody disparate national customs and attitudes about doctor-patient relations but also are relevant to the capacity to ration care in the two nations.

The Private Sector

A budget-limited system, by definition, lacks the resources to provide all care for everyone who is otherwise qualified to receive it. A critical question for those administering budget limits is whether and on what terms to authorize a parallel system through which people with higher-than-average demands for health care or high income can secure more care than the budgeted system provides. Conversely, a critical question for those worried about continued political support for adequate spending in the budgeted system is whether such support erodes when people with high demands for health care can satisfy their wants elsewhere. The British have permitted the private sector to survive as a safety valve but have limited its attractiveness and growth.

Even this small sector is odious to a minority with strongly egalitarian views. They see the private medical care system as atavistic, delivering better care to the economically privileged. To those of a libertarian bent, in contrast, the NHS is the problem. They believe that provision of health care should be determined entirely by individuals operating in free markets, not by bureaucrats or politicians. But for the majority of the British, both Labour and Conservative, the private system provides a useful supplement to the widely embraced National Health Service for selected services and a minority of users.

Aneurin Bevan, the Labour minister who fathered the legislation creating the NHS, overcame the opposition of the medical profession to "socialized medicine" by promising that physicians employed by the NHS could have part-time private practices. Whether Bevan thereby sold the NHS's soul or co-opted the medical profession with a farsighted compromise is still argued. Among the 190,000 acute care beds in NHS hospitals, there are about 3,000 authorized "pay beds" to which consultants may admit private patients. Some pay beds are located in regular NHS wards. A growing number—1,414 in 2001—are located in dedicated private patient units in NHS hospitals.[37] Pay beds work as follows: Hospitals charge private patients for the estimated cost of care. Consultants bill patients separately for their services, as is customary in the United States. Patients or their insurers pay the bill. However payment is arranged, the patient who uses a private bed can circumvent some of the delays or other limits of the NHS.

In 2000, 235 private hospitals in England and Wales had 9,503 beds, 5 percent of all beds. When these are added to the 3,000 NHS pay beds, it makes a total of approximately 12,500 beds for private care.[38] Voluntary insurance covered roughly 80 percent of private admissions for elective hospital treatment in England and Wales in 1997–98, while out-of-pocket payments for private care made up 10.8 percent of all health expenditures in the United Kingdom.[39] British private hospitals have not typically had the range of services available in NHS hospitals—house staff or comprehensive laboratory services, for example—although the capacity of private facilities has steadily improved, and they now perform many advanced procedures. Nonetheless, private hospitals are not the preferred place of treatment for complex or risky surgery or for serious illness.[40]

Private outlays constitute a scant 6 percent of total expenditures on physicians and on inpatient and outpatient care, and account for just under one-fifth of total expenditures.[41] But in particular regions and for specific services, the role of the private medical system is far larger than these fractions suggest. Private medicine is disproportionately located in and around London and the relatively wealthy southwest. Data on the proportion of NHS consultants in various regions who see patients privately support these reports.[42] In 2000 private medical insurance covered 6.9 million people—only 11.5 percent of the population nationwide but a far larger share of professionals and managers.[43] Insurance is an attractive fringe benefit that enables businesses to ensure key employees prompt service for elective care. Privately insured patients thereby avoid queues and other delays common to the NHS. Several unions also have sought health insurance coverage. In the early 1990s, three-fifths of respondents in one survey reported that avoiding NHS waiting lists was a major motivation for seeking private insurance; only 9 percent cited a negative experience with the NHS as an impetus for seeking private care.[44] A fifth of all surgery and 30 percent of hip operations were carried out in the private sector in that year.[45] Just over half of all abortions are done privately, accounting for one admission in nine to private hospitals in 1997–98.[46] The fact that patients can turn to private medicine for abortions and for care of chronic, non-life-threatening conditions means that the NHS can direct its limited resources to treatment of conditions it regards as more urgent.

Private medical insurance is not comprehensive. Individual plans typically do not cover chronic conditions, accidents, or normal pregnancy and childbirth. Some plans explicitly exclude coverage unless NHS waiting lists require waits of more than six weeks.[47] Given these exclusions, premiums are high and have been outpacing cost increases in the National Health Service.[48] Marketing practices have been confusing and misleading. Particularly questionable were so-called moratorium policies, under which preexisting conditions are covered only if the insured receives no medical treatment for those conditions for the first two years of coverage, thereby discouraging treatment of established illnesses.[49]

Patients may enter the private system at various points. A few sign up with private general practitioners. In 2000 only 200 GPs, accounting for only 4 percent of GP consultations, practiced privately in all of England.[50] More often patients elect to see a consultant privately, either directly or after an initial referral by their NHS general practitioner. For example, patients told that they must wait for treatment within the NHS may ask if they can receive treatment more quickly from the consultant as a private patient. Or patients facing a long wait for a bed in an NHS hospital may choose prompt treatment in a private hospital or nursing home. Amenities in private facilities, most of which are new, are often superior to those in NHS hospitals, many of which are old. Yet the smallness of the private sector more than half a century after the creation of the NHS testifies to the reservoir of popular satisfaction with the public system.

The fact that the same consultants who control waiting lists within the NHS also provide similar services privately on a fee-for-service basis not only offers a safety valve for those with insistent demands but also creates the potential for abuses. The field of interventional cardiology is illustrative. If a partially blocked coronary artery is found during an angiogram, it is standard medical practice to perform the indicated angioplasty at the same time. The reason is that the act of threading a catheter into coronary arteries, which is necessary for both for angiography and angioplasty, carries some risk to the patient. Performing both procedures at the same time means that the patient undergoes a risky procedure once, rather than twice. Nevertheless, some NHS cardiologists, who also practice privately, are reported not to perform the angioplasty at the same time that an angiogram identifies a partially occluded artery. Instead, they may inform patients when they regain consciousness that it will be some time before the procedure can be performed within the NHS, but that the procedure can be performed quickly if they are seen as private patients.[51] Similar abuses occur in the United States, where some physicians are also reported to manipulate treatments in order to increase billings.[52]

Premiums for private health insurance remain low by U.S. standards but have been rising rapidly in recent years.[53] Premiums are low in part because almost all patients use their NHS general practitioner, even if they plan to see a consultant privately. In addition, the NHS provides backup protection against serious complications. For example, a patient undergoing hip surgery may elect a private facility because of its availability and amenities. Should a complication arise—a major cardiac or pulmonary problem or a serious infection, for example—the patient can be promptly transferred to a fully equipped and staffed NHS hospital. Furthermore, the population covered by private insurance is usually employed and fairly young, and hence low risk. Finally, British doctors are paid much less than their U.S. counterparts—on the average.[54] However, private rates are unconstrained by NHS salaries, and private charges are far higher than NHS costs.

Whether private medicine should be encouraged, shackled, or put out of existence was once among the most divisive issues facing British society and its policymakers. In 1976, for example, the Labour government began to eliminate pay beds after their numbers had dwindled about 22 percent over the previous decade and their occupancy rates were low.[55] In 1979 the Conservative government reversed that policy. Labour pledged to complete the elimination of private beds in NHS facilities when it returned to power but did not do so.

Now, nearly six decades after the creation of the NHS, a small private sector is accepted by all except a few, largely left-wing members of the Labour party. This acceptance applies not only to privately owned facilities and private physician practices but also to pay beds within National Health Service facilities. Debate has shifted from whether the private sector should exist to whether the government should use private care to shorten the queue of patients compelled to wait long periods for NHS care and use private managers to handle certain NHS facilities. Opportunities for abusive practices by some private physicians will diminish when and if increased NHS spending enables the substantial elimination of lengthy waiting lists.

The sharply ideological character of past debates about the role of the private sector seems to have been replaced with a more pragmatic examination of how the private sector can be used to advance the still widely shared commitment to ensure all residents of Britain health care that is largely free at time of service. But a fundamental issue remains. A private sector provides a "safety valve" for those who are most resistant to budget limits. By "going private," these high-demand patients can escape the consequences of fiscal constraints. The private option may, thereby, abet tighter controls than would otherwise be acceptable. But if private care becomes the norm, the whole purpose of a national health service may be compromised.

The 2005 decision of the Canadian Supreme Court striking down the prohibition of private insurance in Quebec underscores the extreme strategic significance of decisions about whether to allow private-market safety valves and the form they may take. Commentators have raised concerns that this court decision may force wholesale revisions of the health care system throughout Canada.[56]

Conclusions

At least six features of the British health care system have facilitated the imposition of budget limits and made them stick. First, the National Health Service is organized within a parliamentary democracy marked by party discipline. The House of Commons seldom reverses cabinet policy, particularly on budget matters. Second, the Thatcher reforms introduced some elements of market allocation within a budget-constrained system, thereby adapting to a growing restiveness with bureaucratic decision-making. Third, the NHS has retained sequential referral of patients—from general practitioner to consultant. Empowering the GP as gatekeeper creates a mechanism, not widely used in the United States, whereby a trusted family doctor can screen out cases not deemed medically suitable for complex care within prevailing budget limits.[57] Fourth, physicians enjoy a residue of authority, partly based on deference to them as upper-class members of society, which enables them to persuade patients that aggressive treatment is inappropriate and to induce them to accept such bleak news. Fifth, the British are less driven than Americans by the "don't just stand there, do something" attitude toward disease.

Finally, a deep bedrock of support for the egalitarian principles of the National Health Service sustains support for the system, despite limited resources. A leading nephrologist described both the severe resource limits that he encounters and his abiding affection for the National Health Service:

> I usually start off talks by describing the bureaucracy and the rest. And after twenty minutes, people are in tears and inconsolable. But then one can turn it around. And when you've got socialized health care, you've still got intact many of the things that can disappear in a much more brutal system. You've got district nurses driving around visiting people in their own homes, all free. You've got great empowerment of nurse practitioners, because doctors don't have any ownership advantage in owning patients. You get quick referral between primary and secondary care. . . . You get all of these advantages that you can start to list, and then people cheer up and think, "Oh, this is not a bad health care system at all.". . . And having seen the American system, I was quite looking forward to coming back here, actually, strangely enough, to this cash-starved system over here. It seems to me more healthy. And I think we've got to find some way of getting some financial lubrication of this whole system to help us deliver the service, but yet keeping an eye on the holistic aim of what health care is trying to do.

The next three chapters report on how the two health care systems, those of the United States and Great Britain, have managed the availability of a variety of medical technologies and procedures. These chapters explain each medical technology and present information on relative rates of use. This comparison—of procedures that save lives, reduce pain, and improve information—provides data points for inferring the motivations that would be at work when—and if—the United States elects to set limits on spending that force health care rationing.

CHAPTER THREE

Matters of Life and Death

New ways to prevent death constitute some of the most spectacular and costly advances in health care:

—Death from chronic, severe kidney failure was sure and swift until machines were invented that could replace many of the excretory functions of the kidney and ways were found to prevent or slow the failure of kidney transplants.

—Victims of hemophilia, the bleeding disease linked in history texts to royalty, could not be effectively treated until the key blood constituents that produce normal clotting were isolated. Now, hemophilia's devastating symptoms can be treated. Its victims, though never cured, can live almost normally.

—Stem cell transplantation has become a last, best hope for some victims of various otherwise lethal cancers and anemias.

—Intensive care has emerged as one of the most rapidly growing and important functions of the modern hospital, increasing survival among patients, many of whom would have died before its advent.

Understanding how resource limits constrain the availability of these vital services provides a window on the choices rationing forces a nation to make.

Dialysis and Kidney Transplantation

Kidney failure may be temporary or progressive and irreversible. In either case, toxic wastes accumulate in body fluids. A modified diet, especially one low in protein, can slow the dangerous and potentially fatal buildup of such waste products. Acute reversible kidney failure usually results during catastrophic illness, from vascular or septic shock, or from medications. Urine flow diminishes and may stop for a few days or weeks. In such cases, brief dialysis may save a life at relatively low cost. If kidney failure is severe and chronic, however, only long-term renal replacement therapy—dialysis or transplantation—can keep the patient alive. Chronic kidney failure may be sudden or progressive and may result from a wide variety of medical conditions, most notably diabetes.

Dialysis

Dialysis can be performed in two ways. In hemodialysis, blood is allowed to flow from one of the patient's blood vessels via a catheter through a machine in which waste products and excess fluids and salts from the patient's blood diffuse through a thin membrane into a solution, which is then discarded. The cleansed blood is then returned to the patient's circulatory system. This process usually takes four to five hours. It must be repeated regularly, ideally three times a week. In peritoneal dialysis, a special solution is introduced into the abdominal cavity via a flexible plastic tube inserted through the abdominal wall. Waste products, plus excess water and salt, move into the solution by osmosis through the membrane that lines the abdominal cavity. The fluid is periodically drained and replaced with fresh solution. Both procedures take considerable time and may generate nasty side effects.

HEMODIALYSIS. Until the 1960s, hemodialysis could only briefly delay death from irreversible kidney failure. Repeated insertion of a glass tube or cannula progressively destroyed accessible blood vessels so that eventually no way would remain to connect the patient to the dialysis machine. In the early 1960s, a special Teflon shunt connecting artery and vein was developed that could usually be left in place for six months or more.[1] Eventually, complications such as clotting or infection forced its removal. Later a technique was developed to directly connect an artery and a vein and close the skin so that the body surface is left intact. Such a "vascular fistula" functions longer than a shunt does and is less unsightly. Also, graft material such as Goretex or modified bovine veins expanded the options for gaining access to the circulation. These techniques greatly facilitated long-term hemodialysis.

The machines and solutions used in hemodialysis have been improved steadily over the past two decades. New machines with more biocompatible membranes and increased internal surface areas clean the blood faster and more thoroughly than older models did. Although the new membranes have come down in cost, they remain about twice as expensive as the older ones.[2] Improved solutions have also been introduced that reduce the side effects that made dialysis remarkably unpleasant for many patients. They also cut the duration of treatment episodes by about half. But these advances boost costs in two ways: they are more costly per treatment, and they enable more patients to remain on long-term dialysis.

PERITONEAL DIALYSIS. Peritoneal dialysis originally was useful primarily in acute, transient kidney failure. It was not much used in chronic kidney failure because patients had to remain immobile many hours each week and because of various complications, notably infections. Technical improvements have made it possible to use peritoneal dialysis to treat chronic kidney failure. Continuous ambulatory peritoneal dialysis permits the patient to be mobile and can be used by unaided patients. Automated peritoneal dialysis can be performed either in a patient's home or in a medical center while the patient sleeps.

SURVIVAL. Long-term mortality rates among patients undergoing dialysis have fallen but still remain high, typically from comorbidities that originally contributed to renal disease. Mortality on dialysis slightly exceeds that from colon cancer and is only slightly lower than that from lung cancer.[3] In the United States in 1980, the mortality rate during the first year of dialysis was 26 percent. By 1999 first-year mortality had fallen to 23 percent.[4] First-year mortality in the United Kingdom—not adjusted for age or underlying patient health—is almost identical at about 24 percent.[5] These comparisons are difficult to interpret because treatment rates and patient characteristics, notably average age and comorbidities, vary between countries and over time.

Transplantation

Transplantation has a great advantage over dialysis. Successful transplants not only free patients from the travails of dialysis but also give them a sense of good health for as long as the transplanted organ continues to function. Transplantation is feasible, however, only if two conditions are met. First, patients must be able to withstand the rigors of surgery. Second, kidneys must be found that the transplant recipient's body will not reject. Rejection is a natural response to all foreign proteins. It is not a problem if the donor is the recipient's identical twin because the recipient's body will not treat the transplant as "foreign." In all other cases, the recipient must be treated with drugs to prevent or slow graft rejection. Kidneys from living donors (people are born with two kidneys but can live with one) are rejected less quickly than are those from cadavers.

The first drug that effectively reduced rejection of transplants—cyclosporin—became available in 1978.[6] Even with this drug, failure rates were high in 1980. Nearly 40 percent of all kidneys transplanted from cadavers and almost 20 percent of kidneys transplanted from living related donors failed within one year, and cumulative failure rates continued to increase after the first year.[7] Autopsies indicated evidence of damage even in patients whose transplants had not completely failed by the time they died. Patients whose transplants failed either received another one or returned to dialysis.

Many drugs more effective than cyclosporin have since become available. Several others are in the experimental stage or undergoing clinical trials.[8] As a result, transplant failure rates have plummeted. From 1993 through 2002, U.S. one-year graft failure rates averaged 6 percent for transplants from living donors and 11 percent for kidneys from cadavers.[9]

First-year patient mortality after kidney transplantation is similar in the United Kingdom (6 percent and 1 percent, respectively, for cadaver and living donor transplants) and the United States (5 percent and 2 percent, respectively). Transplant rates were higher in the United States than in the United Kingdom—4.5 kidney transplant procedures per 100,000 population were performed in the United States, compared to 2.7 per 100,000 in the United Kingdom.[10] The similarity of mortality rates may therefore be misleading because the higher U.S. transplant rates suggest that sicker U.S. patients may be receiving transplants. The fact that both Canada and Australia, with expenditures between those of the United States and the United Kingdom, had far lower mortality rates underscores the importance of patient selection and other aspects of medical care, factors that have proven impossible to evaluate.[11] (See table 3-1 for a comparison of graft failure and mortality rates in the United Kingdom and Australia.)

A shortage of usable kidneys constrains transplantation in both the United States and Great Britain. Physicians in both nations bewail the failure to harvest potentially transplantable kidneys. Caregivers are loath to bring up the subject of organ donation to terminally ill patients and their families. Transporting kidneys from one area to another is also difficult. The British point to lower murder and traffic fatality rates as an additional reason for a shortage of kidneys. Because the supply of transplantable kidneys is so limited, both countries have lengthy waiting lists

Table 3-1. *Kidney Graft Failure and Mortality Rates,*
United Kingdom and Australia, 1996–99

Percent of transplant patients

Age in years	Graft failure		Patient mortality	
	United Kingdom	Australia	United Kingdom	Australia
25–44	12	7	3	2
45–64	16	11	8	6
65 or older	23	16	17	9

Source: Personal communication from David Ansell, U.K. Renal Registry, Bristol, United Kingdom, November 10, 2003.

for transplants. In 2003 only 28 percent of the 56,621 U.S. patients awaiting kidneys received transplants.[12] In 2003–04 roughly 300 patients in the United Kingdom and 3,700 in the United States died before a kidney became available.[13]

Cost of Treatment

Dialysis costs averaged $52,000 a year per patient in 2001 in the United States.[14] Adjusted for inflation, that price has changed little for the past two decades.[15] In Great Britain the cost of hemodialysis in 2000–01 was about three fifths as high—$31,713 in hospitals; $27,717 at home; and $30,299 in dedicated dialysis centers, usually attached to hospitals.[16] At least part of the cost difference doubtlessly stems from disparities in compensation of physicians, nurses, and technicians.

Kidney transplants are far more costly in the United States than in Britain—$95,000 to $115,000 versus an estimated $20,983.[17] The data on graft failure and patient mortality could be interpreted as indicating that the United States is not buying improved outcomes with its higher outlays; but, once again, these data do not control for comorbidities and other factors that influence patient outcomes.

Financial Influences

Dialysis, like all other health care services, is free to the British patient. Since 1972 the End Stage Renal Disease (ESRD) program has covered most costs for U.S. patients and pays physicians or dialysis centers a fee that covers costs and profit. But the two payment methods differ in a crucial respect. The British give dialysis centers an annually fixed budget that does not vary within the year according to the number of patients served. Treating more patients does not increase center revenue. To the extent that center staff persuade patients to accept home dialysis or a transplant, more resources are left for those still requiring dialysis. The ESRD program, in contrast, pays U.S. dialysis centers a fee for each patient served. It rewards dialysis centers for adding to their patient lists but not for encouraging patients to take home dialysis or a transplant.

British nephrologists speculate that these incentives may encourage nephrologists to prescribe peritoneal dialysis in Britain, even when patients lack the support necessary to carry it out effectively. They also think fixed annual budgets may have caused centers to put more people on home dialysis than is medically optimal. Home dialysis places considerable demands of time and skill on patients and their families, many of whom are not equipped to handle this demanding mode of therapy. The method of payment may also have led British nephrologists to advise transplants in patients unlikely to have good outcomes.[18]

Fixed annual National Health Service (NHS) budgets mean that managers of British dialysis centers must compete with other health services for funding and personnel. Hospital dialysis faces the additional challenge of having to compete for limited hospital space. Consultant nephrologists must secure hospital space, dialysis machines, and permission to hire and train nurses and technicians to run them. A lack of machines at one time restricted dialysis, but equipment is now less of a bottleneck than personnel. Implementing a home dialysis program was easier than starting or enlarging a center. It required no scarce hospital space. It took only enough nursing time to train patients and their families but did not require skilled nursing personnel for day-to-day supervision. Once a patient is trained, the principal direct costs for continued home dialysis are for fluids and other sterile supplies. Even during the lean years, when NHS budgets barely kept pace with inflation, the British commitment to clinical freedom meant that each doctor could draw relatively freely on such supplies. Nephrologists could increase the resources effectively at their disposal by encouraging patients to do home dialysis.[19]

Nephrologists now report that they have more resources, but only because they and various groups of patients have lobbied and politicked incessantly. They tell of going "hat in hand" each year to maintain and increase budgets. They recount a "highest priority" struggle over the "last twenty years . . . to increase the proportion of patients with end stage renal failure who could be treated." In this fight, they see themselves as buttressed by patients, individually and collectively:

> If your patient has coronary artery disease and is thought to require an intervention [and] that intervention is unavailable . . . they will not be dead three weeks on Friday. . . . But the pressure that dialysis gives us is being able to say [that] this patient is going to die in three weeks unless we dialyze them. . . . The great thing about renal patients is that you are a renal patient for life. [They say] "Look at me. This is my life. I've been on dialysis for ten years, and I have had two transplants. So don't tell me I don't know what is going on." And they are incredibly powerful.

Nephrologists do not claim that this struggle has eliminated rationing, only that effort has reduced it. Current treatment levels are sustainable with available resources, they say, only because staff work more hours than they are paid for and quality is compromised in various ways. Furthermore, they foresee worse to come as caseloads are expected to explode.

Frequency

A quarter century ago, the difference between rates of treatment for chronic renal failure in the United States and Great Britain was huge (see table 3-2).[20] In the early 1980s, few British chronic renal failure patients over the age of fifty or fifty-five were dialyzed or received transplants. Compared to their colleagues in France, West Germany, and Italy, British nephrologists treated new patients through age forty-four at the same rate, but older patients at progressively lower rates. Patients with vascular complications of diabetes were considered unsuitable for treatment in Britain.

These dry facts represent a grisly reality—many middle-aged and elderly British patients with renal failure, who could have been treated and lived, went untreated and died. Perhaps even more striking was evidence that many British physicians told their patients—and themselves—that they and the National Health Service were providing optimal care.

Not only the level, but also the mix of treatment differed between the United States and Great Britain. U.S. hemodialysis rates were more than three times those in Britain. The new technology of peritoneal dialysis, little used in the early 1980s, was introduced faster in Britain because it was cheaper and freed up costly dialysis machines or scarce hospital or center

Table 3-2. *Rates of Treatment for Renal Failure, United States and United Kingdom*

Number of procedures per million population

Mode of treatment	1980 U.S.[a]	1980 U.K.[b]	2002 U.S.[a]	2002 U.K.
Hemodialysis	190	60	978	244
Peritoneal dialysis	3	9	86	92
Functioning transplant	42	56	424	289
Total	249	128	1,496	625

Sources: U.S. Renal Data System online database and *2004 Annual Data Report* (http://www.usrds.org/adr.htm (June 2005); C. Jacobs and others, "Combined Report on Regular Dialysis and Transplantation in Europe, XI, 1970," *Proceedings of the European Dialysis and Transplant Association* 18 (1981): 4–58; David Ansell and others, eds., *U.K. Renal Registry Report 2003* (Bristol, U.K.: U.K. Renal Registry, December 2003).

a. U.S. totals for 1980 and 2002 include 14 and 8 cases per million, respectively, whose mode of treatment was unknown.

b. U.K. total for 1980 includes 3 cases per million whose mode of treatment was unknown.

beds. Transplants were performed at almost the same rate in Britain as in the United States, but a larger proportion of those treated in Britain than in the United States remained alive with functioning grafts, perhaps because the patients selected for therapy were in better average health.

In the succeeding two decades, treatment of renal failure increased enormously in both countries. In Britain treatment rates in 2002 were nearly five times the rate in 1980 and more than twice what they had been in the United States in 1980. Nearly one-third of British dialysis patients were receiving peritoneal dialysis, compared with less than one-tenth in the United States.[21] The number of patients with functioning transplants had risen dramatically in both countries, but more rapidly in the United States (see table 3-2). Even more striking was the decline of age-based rationing in Britain. In 1980 few people over age fifty and almost none over age sixty were dialyzed in Great Britain. In 2002 nearly half of new patients being accepted for renal replacement therapy in the United Kingdom were age sixty-five or over, roughly the same fraction as in the United States.[22]

Limitations on Treatment: A Puzzle

The data in table 3-2 pose an intriguing puzzle. Everyone now agrees that dialysis was rationed in Great Britain in the early 1980s. The virtual absence of patients over the age of fifty-five makes rationing hard to deny. At the same time, U.S. nephrologists believed that they were treating all suitable candidates. Indeed, the ESRD program was enacted in part to spare physicians and the nation the moral anguish and psychological distress entailed in deciding which patients with renal failure should be treated—and live—and which should be given only comfort therapy— and die.

Two decades later, the British were treating renal failure at more than twice the U.S. rate of 1980. But U.S. treatment rates had increased by a factor of six. Does the fact that the United States was treating patients at more than twice the British rate in 2002 mean that the British are still rationing? Or are U.S. physicians and dialysis centers grossly overtreating? Besides, if the British in 2002 were treating at more than twice the U.S. rate of the 1980s—when, by common agreement, care was not rationed in the United States—how could the British be said to be rationing care?

SOME POSSIBLE SOLUTIONS. In the early 1980s renal failure patients were rejected in both countries because of age and comorbidities that are no longer considered bars to treatment. One veteran British nephrologist recently noted, as evidence that diabetics in the past were denied care for renal failure, that he did not know of any diabetic whose cause of death in the distant past was listed as kidney failure, even though nephropathy is one of the most common and lethal consequences of diabetes. Other somatic diseases, mental illness, and physical handicaps also led to rejection for treatment. People infected with hepatitis were also viewed unfavorably because they had to be treated in segregated areas at great additional expense.

Because distance from therapy deters use, many British patients were effectively denied care because of the paucity of dialysis centers in Great Britain.[23] Most dialysis units were located in academic centers. As a result, one nephrologist reported that Greater London had eleven centers within five miles of one another, while the rest of the country had only forty-four.

The availability of hospital- or center-based dialysis has since been increased. Starting in the 1980s the NHS began to build dialysis centers outside teaching hospitals. As a result, an increasing proportion of potential patients lives within reasonable travel time of a center. Still, NHS funds to build facilities remain sparse. To meet demand, some private investors are building facilities, usually but not always with prior approval of the NHS. Such private investment actually serves the interests of the NHS because it enables increased capacity without requiring an enlarged budget. Still, reports persist that patients are inappropriately shunted into or forced to remain on home dialysis.[24] Convenient location is also an issue in transplants. Expert opinion holds that twenty additional renal transplant units, in addition to the twenty-eight units now operating in the United Kingdom, would be required to treat all suitable candidates.[25]

In the end, however, the questions persist: Why have treatment rates risen so much in both nations? And does the undiminished gap between their treatment rates show unabated rationing?

WHY HAVE TREATMENT RATES RISEN SO MUCH? Several factors contribute to increased treatment rates for renal failure. First, selection criteria for dialysis have become less stringent in both countries, in part because improved technology has shortened dialysis times and reduced side effects. Second, mortality rates among dialysis patients have fallen. Improved quality of life while on dialysis means that patients survive longer on therapy and are less likely to withdraw from treatment and accept death rather than continue a burdensome regime. Third, dialysis and kidney transplantation were relatively new therapies two decades ago. Too little time had passed for patient rolls to grow and reach equilibrium levels. For each of these reasons, the ranks of the successfully treated now include growing numbers of long-term patients and the elderly.[26]

Finally, the epidemiology of renal failure is changing—and quite ominously. In particular, obesity—a risk factor for diabetes—has become epidemic in the United States and is on the rise in Great Britain. Poorly controlled diabetes often leads to renal failure. The prevalence of diabetes in the United States is more than twice that in England.[27] Twenty years ago, diabetics with renal failure were considered terminal and were rarely accepted for renal replacement therapy. Now, an estimated 46 percent of patients accepted for dialysis in the United States and 18 percent in Great Britain are diabetic.[28] Diabetic nephropathy is particularly common among African Americans, Indians, and Pakistanis. Although African Americans form only 13 percent of the U.S. population, they account for 30–35 percent of the dialysis population.[29] British nephrologists also report that most Africans immigrated to Great Britain during the 1970s when conditions were lethal in Uganda and Kenya and "haven't really started aging yet." Thus demographic facts portend a sharp long-term increase in renal failure.

Current trends indicate that the number of U.S. patients with renal failure will double between 2004 and 2010. The British also anticipate that caseloads will rise, doubling over the next decade; if treatment resources are available, that projection could be low.[30]

HAS RATIONING ABATED? International comparative data show that treatment rates in Britain remain small compared to those in the United States and Japan—particularly among the very old—and at least somewhat below those of most other comparable nations.[31] For example, the population-adjusted treatment rate in the United States is roughly three times higher than in the United Kingdom among patients twenty-five to forty-four, but roughly five times higher among patients aged forty-five to eighty-four, and nine times higher among patients age eighty-five or older.[32] One expert put the matter unequivocally: "I think there is clearly bedside rationing of new patients presenting with end stage renal failure. . . . Judgments are made on the spot whether somebody is likely to survive. And some of the sickest people never get treated. That's probably more common in this country than certainly it is in the United States, where I think it's skewed in the other direction." Nephrologists acknowledge that the quality and frequency of care still vary widely across Great Britain. They acknowledge that problems of the past—too few patients on center-based hemodialysis, too many on home dialysis, and too many on peritoneal dialysis—also persist.[33]

As the number of dialysis centers has grown, a seemingly unrelated shortage has created a serious quality issue. Nephrologists in some parts of Britain report that it is difficult to induce vascular surgeons to implant vascular fistulas—the devices that directly link a vein and an artery and permit very long term dialysis with little risk of infection or destruction of vascular access.[34] This problem has arisen, paradoxically, because the number of dialysis centers has increased. When dialysis was confined to teaching hospitals, salaried vascular surgeons were generally available on staff. Regulations prohibit faculty-based consultants from seeing private patients. Thus vascular surgeons were shielded from the temptation to engage in highly remunerated private practice. With the spread of dialysis to district hospitals, which often do not have staff vascular surgeons, nephrologists have found that they must depend, as one nephrologist put the matter with some bitterness,

on the grace and favor of willing general surgeons and willing vascular surgeons who were prepared to spend a little bit of time helping out the renal unit. . . . And you can't get vascular surgeons in the NHS to . . . spend a lot of time with renal patients. . . . Our surgeons work for the National Health Service. But the main part of their salary is in private practice. And, you know, surgeons are tied up and busy people. . . . You don't see many poor surgeons in England, you know. They all drive extremely nice cars, but it's not earned from the National Health Service. It's earned from private practice. . . . We've got a rotten vascular surgery service, and half our patients are on dialysis catheters, where we know that three quarters, at least, should be having fistulas.

Nephrologists also complain that patients would fare better if they were seen earlier in the course of their disease than is now common. Uncontrolled high blood pressure, resulting from obesity or other factors, gradually degrades kidney function. Methods of controlling hypertension are quite effective in delaying the progress of chronic kidney disease. British general practitioners report that screening examinations, for high blood pressure or other conditions, are uncommon. The lack of information from such examinations is a source of concern to nephrologists who believe that a future epidemic of renal failure could be attenuated if patients with incipient problems were screened and treated early.[35]

This problem is not confined to Great Britain. The Medicare Payment Advisory Commission reports that many U.S. renal failure patients are not seen early enough in the course of therapy and that, once seen, many do not receive appropriate screening.[36] Early treatment and frequent screening improve outcomes because kidney failure is a progressive disease.

ATTITUDES—THEN AND NOW. In the early 1980s, some British nephrologists acknowledged rationing as a fact. Others elaborately rationalized their behavior as medically optimal. And still others questioned whether rationing was going on at all. Asked how he would explain to her family the prospects of a sixty-five-year-old woman with kidney failure, one general practitioner first said that he did not think it was up to him to decide whether she should be dialyzed and that he would leave the decision to the consultant. But then he added, "Obviously the patient is sixty-five and therefore does not come within the regional dialysis program." When pressed on whether he might save everyone time and anguish by discouraging referral, he described how he would talk to the family. "I would say that mother's or aunt's kidneys have failed or are failing and there is very little that anybody can do about it because of her age and general physical state, and that it would be my suggestion or my advice that we spare her any further investigation, any further painful procedure, and we would just make her as comfortable as we can for what remains of her life."[37] Remarkably, few of the criteria for rejection were explicitly stated. Age, for example, was never officially identified as a contraindication to treatment.[38]

Despite low treatment rates, nephrologists said that they did not, *and would not*, turn patients away. The Medical Services Study Group of the Royal College of Physicians, from an extensive audit of records of patients under fifty, reported in *The British Medical Journal* in 1981 that no patient was denied dialysis because of inadequate facilities.[39] Most dialysis unit directors reported in 1980 that they were "coping with demand," and British nephrologists claimed that they treated all comers.[40] The task of denying care fell largely to general practitioners and consultants in fields other than nephrology.[41] Local physicians who flouted these norms and referred "unsuitable" patients forced nephrologists to tell patients and their families that treatment was unavailable or to find space where none really existed. If patients were denied care, referring physicians would have had to admit to error in the referral or acknowledge that resource constraints precluded treatment. Little wonder that local internists learned to strike a balance between medical indications and resource realities.

RATIONALIZATION. In the past some British physicians persuaded themselves that decisions forced upon them by a lack of resources were actually medically optimal. When asked to explain why sixty-year-old patients with renal failure but no other complicating conditions, in full possession of their faculties, and productive at work or home should be denied care, one nephrologist reported that he heard that a basis for rejections was that "the patient spoke no English."[42] A contemporary nephrologist expressed outrage and said that in more than two decades of practice he had never heard such a justification for failure to treat and believed that it would not occur. Whether a contemporary nephrologist was accurately commenting on cultural differences or repeating the earlier bias was not clear when he told us,

I think there is no doubt that . . . in different . . . cultural groups . . . there are very major differences in attitudes toward death and illness. . . . Roughly 40 percent of patients [in London] on our end stage renal failure programs . . . came from the Indian subcontinent.

And many people from that culture . . . feel that it was inappropriate to, if you like, move against the forces of—greater forces, shall
we say. Now that obviously doesn't happen to the fully westernized
people. But it illustrates that many people, [if you] tell them that
they have end stage renal failure, fine. If you can do something,
[they are] not interested.

One English consultant in 1980 justified failure to treat the elderly
because everyone over fifty-five is "a bit crumbly" and therefore not
really a suitable candidate for therapy. In 2004 another nephrologist, who
had just said that age would never *by itself* justify denial of therapy and
who had just been told of the remark that people over age fifty were "a
bit crumbly," said, "Well, actually that is factually correct." Nonetheless,
surveys indicate that British nephrologists and others disapprove of age-
based rationing as frequently as do Americans.[43]

Constraints on availability of care have been relaxed but not eliminated. The number of dialysis centers has increased, and the prevalence of
treatment has more than quadrupled. But nephrologists continue to
bemoan a lack of resources and the grinding need to continually scrounge
for funds. They also point to huge geographic variations in the frequency
and quality of treatment.[44] Although NHS budgets have risen, they
remain more limited than the almost unconstrained U.S. system of paying
for treatment of renal failure. Cost remains a factor in certain aspects of
treatment in Great Britain, but much more subtly than in the past. For
example, transplants of kidneys from living donors have become common in the United States, partly because of the development of laparo-
scopic donor nephrectomy—a procedure in which a donor's kidney can
be removed through a small incision. This procedure reduces risk to
donors and speeds their recovery relative to older procedures that used
large incisions. The newer procedure is not widely available in the United
Kingdom because it is expensive and requires more total surgical time
than the transplantation of cadaver kidneys.[45] A lack of intensive care
beds has also contributed to the paucity of kidney donations from living
donors in Great Britain.[46] Transplantable kidneys were also in short supply in the United States, where the transplant rate also fell during the
1990s and waiting lists grew by 50 percent.[47]

U.S. nephrologists would probably treat renal failure more aggressively than their British colleagues, even if resources were suddenly equal-
ized. Conversely, conservative physician attitudes in Britain, based on

years of practice under stringent conditions, would not suddenly turn aggressive if resource limits vanished. Nor would U.S. physicians placidly accept constraints that British physicians regard as part of the medical climate. As one British physician put the matter,

> If physicians over here had infinite resources, they would treat person-for-person less people here than you would treat in the United States or in mainland Europe. . . . I think there is a different attitude to end stage renal failure here. . . . Dialysis is not that great a treatment for high-risk patients, many of whom are dying in any case from multiple comorbid conditions. . . . And we have an active program of supporting people in end stage renal failure without dialysis. That doesn't mean they are neglected. They are given all of the infrastructure support that dialysis patients get. . . . And, so, not all patients go onto dialysis. One could argue for good reason. I think it's just an example of modern interventional technology being misused. . . .
>
> I'd put much more resources into end of life management, into palliative care, skilled palliative care facilities, proper facilities for care of the dying. And proper relationships with the holistic care that hospices can buy. In other words, I'd recognize end stage renal failure as a legitimate cause of death, and it's got to be managed as such, not complicated by an uncritical application of dialysis.

A U.S. physician echoed the latter sentiment in pointing out the need not just to provide dialysis but to provide end of life and palliative care for the population already on dialysis but displeased with their quality of life. The fastest growing cause of death among dialysis patients in the United States is voluntary withdrawal from therapy.[48]

Hemophilia

While U.S. and British treatments of renal failure differ widely, both nations handle hemophilia similarly. Three factors seem to be of particular importance. The first is aggregate cost. Optimal treatment per patient can be enormously costly, but the number of hemophiliacs is small. As a result, the aggregate cost has been low enough that even a budget-constrained system, such as that of Great Britain, can afford full care. The second is the nature of the disease. Undertreated hemophiliacs suffer visibly and painfully and generate large additional costs. With modern therapy hemophiliacs enjoy close to normal life expectancies. In contrast, undertreated renal failure patients vanish quietly—they simply die. The third factor is age: hemophilia is typically diagnosed in children, while chronic renal failure usually strikes the middle-aged and old.

Nature of the Disease

Hemophilia, the bleeding disease associated in popular lore with royal families, is usually genetic in origin. Women carry the defective gene. They transmit it, on the average, to half their daughters, who suffer no symptoms but transmit it, on the average, to half their sons, who suffer from the disease. Hemophilia occurs in approximately 1 in every 4,000 live male births.

Hemophilia is a single name for two diseases characterized by the partial or complete absence of either of two blood components. Patients with hemophilia A lack factor VIII; those with hemophilia B lack factor IX. Both factors are necessary for normal clotting. Apparently no one suffers from both variants of the disease. Hemophilia may be classified as severe, moderate, or mild, according to the proportion of the normal endowment of factor VIII or factor IX that is missing. Somewhat over half of all hemophiliacs suffer from a severe form of the disease.[49]

The disease usually becomes apparent in childhood, although mild hemophilia may not be diagnosed until later in the patient's life, when some event, such as surgery, uncovers the condition. Contrary to popular myth, the scourge of hemophiliacs is not fatal hemorrhage after a small cut or bruise. Rather, nonfatal internal hemorrhages occur periodically, either spontaneously or following minor trauma. Severe untreated hemophiliacs average about two bleeding episodes a month. Frequency depends on whether the patient produces some or none of each factor and on age, activities, and previous treatment.[50]

An episode begins with a feeling of tingling or warmth and may be accompanied by restlessness or anxiety. Within a few hours, the patient may experience mild discomfort and restriction of motion. Next come pain, swelling, skin warmth, and severe limits on motion. The blood that caused the symptoms is eventually resorbed over periods ranging from days to weeks.

Bleeding usually occurs in joints. Each episode damages, and repeated bleeding may destroy, the joint in which it occurs. Sometimes bleeds occur in muscles or the kidneys, and, in rare but dangerous cases, the head. Seriously affected patients suffer devastating and painful episodes which, if untreated, occur with increasing frequency and lead to disability and early death—at age eleven, on the average, before the advent of modern treatment methods.[51]

Patients may be treated "prophylactically"—that is, given the missing factor on a regular schedule to reduce the likelihood of a bleeding episode—or "on demand"—after a bleed has occurred. Patients who are treated prophylactically still develop bleeds; accordingly, some patients are treated in both ways. In either case, treatment is most effective if begun in the patient's infancy and, if on demand, at the earliest moment after onset of a bleed to palliate short-term discomfort and minimize long-term damage.

History of Treatment

The history of hemophilia treatment is a drama in three acts: medical breakthrough, tragedy, and recovery.

Until the late 1960s, hemophilia could be treated only with cumbersome transfusions of plasma from healthy blood donors. Such treatment boosted life expectancy from eleven to twenty years. The problem with such transfusions is that each unit of normal plasma contains little factor VIII or factor IX. The maximum volume of transfused fluids patients could tolerate does not contain enough of the missing blood factor to forestall frequent hospitalization and progressive damage.

During the second half of the 1960s, techniques were developed to reduce the volume of each transfusion. If plasma is frozen and slowly thawed, a cryoprecipitate remains that contains much higher concentrations of factor VIII than plasma does. As a result, it became possible to administer large quantities of factor VIII in a small volume. This advance revolutionized the treatment of hemophilia A. Unfortunately, the cryoprecipitate contains no factor IX, so treatment of hemophilia B was unaffected.

Each unit of cryoprecipitate came from a single donor, but hemophiliacs typically received many units. In the 1970s, partially purified concentrates containing factor VIII and factor IX became available. These products were derived from the plasma of hundreds of donors. Little of the new blood product was initially produced, and only large medical centers had it. By the early 1970s, however, concentrates of factor VIII became readily available in both the United States and Britain. By the mid-1970s nearly all patients were entered into treatment programs. That the new concentrates did not have to be kept frozen also facilitated home therapy. Life expectancy jumped to sixty-four years in 1983.[52]

In a horrifying turn of events, shortly after factor concentrates became available and widely used, scientists first recognized human immunodeficiency virus (HIV). They also realized that blood donations had become infected with HIV and hepatitis. Because factor concentrates were produced from pooled blood donations, the "wonderful" new method of treating hemophilia had become an infernally efficient way of infecting victims of one life-threatening condition with another lethal disease. By the early 1980s, 60 to 70 percent of severe hemophiliacs in Western Europe and the United States were HIV positive.[53] Life expectancy plummeted to forty years.[54] To compound this misfortune, many also were infected with hepatitis.

The infection of hemophiliacs with HIV led to new techniques of treating factor concentrates that dramatically reduced the risk of viral transmission.[55] New genetically engineered products were developed using recombinant-DNA technology that drastically reduced the risk of infection and also ended progressive liver damage resulting from previously available blood products.[56] The gene for producing factor VIII or factor IX is spliced into genes from mammalian cells in tissue culture, which then generate the factor as cells divide and multiply. Clotting factors produced by these methods became available in the early 1990s. They have only two drawbacks: they cost two to three times as much as human-blood-derived products, and production is difficult, making them available only in limited quantities.[57]

Dose

When a patient suffers a bleeding episode, administration of factor VIII or factor IX normally ends the bleeding and associated discomfort. The aim of treatment is to increase the naturally missing blood factor enough to permit healing and prevent further bleeds, at least for a while. The duration of treatment and the success and speed of recovery depend on where the bleed occurs and how much damage was done, the severity of the underlying disease, the age and previous treatment of the patient, the speed with which medication is administered after the onset of an episode, and the patient's healing time.[58] The duration of treatment ranges from a day or two to two weeks or more. The World Health Organization estimates that average adults require 28,000 to 105,000 units of factor VIII annually if treated on demand, but from 110,000 to 427,000 units if treated prophylactically.[59] However, large doses are thought to increase somewhat the risk of abnormal liver function resulting from impurities in the blood samples from which the factors are obtained.[60] Thus the clinically optimal dosage for on-demand treatment is subject to a wide range of variability and some uncertainty. Furthermore, among U.S. patients, approximately 15 percent of those with severe hemophilia A and 2.5 percent of all those with hemophilia B develop inhibitory antibodies to the coagulation factors. This complication necessitates very large and costly doses of "bypassing" agents and factor VIIa (a recombinant version of clotting factor VII) to overcome resistance.[61] The corresponding proportions of patients with such antibodies in the United Kingdom are quite similar, at 14 percent and 1 percent, respectively.[62]

Therapeutic Standards

A critical therapeutic question concerns how much of the deficient factor patients should receive. Two decades ago, the average U.S. patient received about 50 percent more factor VIII concentrate or cryoprecipitate than did the average British patient. Despite these differences, all diagnosed patients in both countries were treated to levels physicians thought optimal. Few studies of the consequences of different dosages had then been done. Early work seemed to indicate that doses even lower than those then used in Britain would produce satisfactory results. But in 1980 one study by a British team indicated that doses approximating those then common in the United States were often more effective than smaller doses, though lower doses sometimes suffice. Accordingly, the difference between British and U.S. dosages lay within the range of clinical uncertainty. Although British physicians favored a less intensive, lower-cost program of therapy than American practice, they claimed that medical considerations, not resource limits, dictated how they practiced.

Current national data on the average dosage are scarce, but treatment methods seem to have converged. One crude indicator of dose levels can be derived by dividing total sales of clotting factors by national population.[63] Based on this approach, usage of factor VIII is nearly identical in the United States and the United Kingdom—3.4 and 3.29 units per person, respectively.[64] As before, physicians seem to be following the dictates of medical judgment, not of budget limits, in the treatment of hemophilia.

The nature of insurance coverage in the United States may influence therapy, however. Just under two-thirds of U.S. hemophiliacs in one survey used some kind of factor concentrate in 1998, and just over one-third used none. Of nonusers, 70 percent were insured by commercial insurers and 26 percent by Medicare or Medicaid. Of the users, 51 percent were insured by commercial insurers and 45 percent by Medicare and Medicaid.

Cost

Therapeutic cost depends on both dosage and unit price of factor VIII or factor IX. The average annual cost per patient of treating severe, moderate, and mild hemophilia in the United States is, respectively, more than $100,000, $26,000 to $50,000, and $2,000.[65] The cost of treating patients who have developed antibodies can be staggering. A variety of protocols have been used to reduce or eliminate patients' blood components that inhibit factor VIII from working. All entail prolonged administration of high doses of the missing factor and, usually, additional immunosuppressive treatment. The British report average costs of such patients at approximately £500,000—more than $900,000 at mid-2004 exchange rates. One British health authority recently devoted nearly £2 million—more than $3.2 million over one year—to provide "high-dose" immune tolerance induction to a single boy with severe inhibitors.[66] The debate over whether to provide such treatment clearly highlights the conflicts that can arise between rights-based and utilitarian-based principles of healthcare provision. Suffice it to say that the financial demands of hemophilia have increased and now pose serious challenges to the provision of treatment.

The per patient cost of treatment has risen substantially for three distinct reasons. First, the price of standard blood-derived products has risen. Second, the price of recombinant DNA products is higher than that of blood-derived products. Third, standards of treatment now call for larger doses. In particular, the proportion of patients given prophylactic treatment has risen sharply. Two decades ago, prophylaxis was used in fewer than 5 percent of all cases in the United States and Great Britain. From 1998 to 2002, 23 percent received prophylaxis; for patients with severe hemophilia A, the proportion was 37 percent, with even higher rates among adolescents.[67] National data on prophylaxis in the United Kingdom are unavailable. However, British experts note that since the early 1990s, long-term prophylaxis has been used "whenever feasible" to treat British children with severe hemophilia and for all one- to two-year-olds.[68]

The U.S. hemophiliac population was an estimated 19,800 in 2002. The total cost of treatment was approximately $2.7 billion in 2002, of which 97 percent went for the treatment of approximately 13,000 severe hemophiliacs. In the United Kingdom in 2001, the total hemophiliac population was around 6,300, about 2,300 of whom were deemed severely affected. More than 90 percent of the estimated £162 million cost of care for hemophilia went to treatment of severely affected patients.[69] These costs are bound to increase sharply in both countries. The catastrophic HIV epidemic of the 1980s and 1990s means that the current population of hemophiliacs is quite young. Because optimal treatment now promises hemophiliacs a normal life expectancy and new hemophilia victims are born every day, the number of patients under treatment—and the cost of treating them—will grow for decades.

Stem Cell Transplantation

Physicians made medical history in 1968 when they successfully transplanted bone marrow cells from a healthy girl into the bloodstream of her brother, whose body was incapable of producing white blood cells. Because his condition made the boy susceptible to infection, he was spending his life confined to a sterile tent. The transplant succeeded and the boy could leave the tent.[70] Thus began bone marrow transplantation (BMT), a new procedure that was initially used in treating just a few diseases—aplastic anemia, some forms of leukemia, and certain rare inborn errors of metabolism and uncommon deficiencies of the body's immune system.

At first, the British used the procedure at rates comparable to those in the United States. Over time, applications of this procedure have increased and costs have risen. British use of the procedure has begun to lag that in the United States. This lag in spending on what has become a major health outlay is not surprising. A budget-constrained system could provide a little-used, high-prestige service at high rates because the overall cost was trivial. Now that the service has become more widely applicable and the total cost of full care has become burdensome, budget limits are forcing trade-offs.

The Procedure

Normal bone marrow generates red and white blood cells and platelets. Several conditions prevent the body from producing these vital cells. Aplastic anemia, for example, affects roughly 1,000 patients a year in the United States. It was among the first conditions to be treated with bone marrow transplantation. The disease causes the bone marrow to stop or almost stop making some or all white and red blood cells and platelets.[71] The patient then becomes anemic, vulnerable to severe hemorrhage and serious infection. Initial treatment often consists of transfusions of red blood cells or platelets. Transfusing white cells is impractical because white cells survive less than a day on the average. Therefore, those patients whose anemia is characterized by insufficient white cells may receive antibiotics to ward off infection. In mild cases, transfusions of red cells or platelets may sustain the patient for some time, and occasionally, the bone marrow recovers spontaneously. However, only one patient in five survives more than two years when treatment is solely based on transfusions. In contrast, 60 to 90 percent of patients who receive a bone marrow transplant are cured of the disease.[72]

Bone marrow transplants involve transfusing cells from healthy donors into sick patients. Without further steps, however, the recipient's body would treat the infused bone marrow as foreign protein and destroy it. For BMT to succeed, it was essential somehow to stop this rejection. Extreme measures were used to prevent rejection. Large doses of cytotoxic drugs, often combined with total body irradiation, completely suppressed the patient's immune system.[73] For two to three weeks, before the graft begins to function, transfusions of red blood cells and platelets are necessary to prevent fatal anemia, and, because transfer of white blood cells to fight infection is impractical, patients often had to be isolated in sterile rooms and dosed heavily with antibiotics.

Preventing rejection is easier if donor and patient are genetically similar. That is why the bubble boy received a transplant from his sister. Only in 1973, five years after this initial success, did doctors perform the first "allogenic" (from one unrelated human to another) BMT. Six key antigens of donor and recipient had to match. Nonetheless, the patient's body often destroyed the donated marrow (graft rejection), and when the graft began to generate the missing cells, the donated marrow often attacked the patient's own cells, so-called graft-versus-host disease. Twenty-five to 50 percent of patients in the 1980s experienced graft-versus-host disease, and one quarter of them died from that cause.[74] Others contracted severe pneumonia, which also was sometimes fatal. Patients who cleared these hurdles were usually cured and could return to a normal life. Even then, however, some developed chronic graft-versus-host disease or suffered cataracts, sterility, or new cancers caused by the total body irradiation that made BMT effective in the first place.

Bone marrow transplantation unequivocally increased survival of victims of aplastic anemia, as documented in clinical trials, but few patients over age forty initially were treatable. Evidence on its efficacy in treating leukemia and inherited disorders has become available only recently.

Advances

The procedure has been rechristened stem cell therapy (SCT) because the relevant stem cells may be gathered outside bone marrow from the circulating blood. Several other major advances have increased the number of conditions that can be treated and the age of patients who can undergo the procedure. SCT is now used in treating multiple myeloma, some non-hematologic malignant tumors, lymphoma, sickle cell disease, thalassemia, and even autoimmune diseases.[75] The patient's age remains relevant to whether SCT is a recommended therapy, but the procedure is now used in patients as old as age seventy.

Among the most important advances has been the development of techniques enabling patients to serve as their own cell donors. Such "autologous transplantation" became available in 1990s, after the development of new techniques to freeze and store bone marrow cells. Rather than drilling into a patient's bone, clinicians learned to collect transplantable stem cells circulating in the blood. Most autografts now use such "peripheral" blood cells.[76] With this approach the transfused stem cells start working faster than with the older methods. Gathering cells from circulating blood is easier than drilling through bone to harvest bone marrow and avoids contamination with various impurities present in bone marrow. In addition, hospital stays are shorter when circulating cells rather than marrow cells are used.[77]

Autologous procedures have increased the pool of potential transplant recipients. Because the transplant recipient is the donor, autografts disrupt the patient's immune system less than conventional BMT. Autografts are widely used to treat patients with certain types of hematological cancers, including multiple myeloma, lymphoma, and neuroblastoma.[78] Self-donor procedures have also made SCT available to patients with diseases not treatable easily or at all with allogenic procedures.

A recently developed technique dispenses with the radiation or drugs to kill off all of a patient's diseased cells, a procedure that also destroys the patient's immune system. Such nonmyeloablative or so-called mini-transplants can be used in elderly or extremely sick patients who cannot tolerate the intense radiation and chemotherapy used in conventional

SCT. Between 1997 and 2002, 3,000 minitransplants were performed in patients over age fifty; of these, 66 were done in patients older than seventy. This procedure is new and has not yet been fully evaluated.[79]

In 1989, for the first time, stem cells were collected from the blood of a neonate's umbilical cord. In the succeeding fifteen years, about 700 successful transplants using cells from this type of source were performed, typically in children.[80] While the procedure is uncommon, it has the potential to dramatically expand the pool of potential stem cell donations.

Indications for stem cell transplants have expanded dramatically. Clinical trials have confirmed the benefits of SCT for treating some forms of leukemia and several other diseases.[81] The age ceiling on allogenic grafts has risen from about forty to the sixties, and for autologous grafts, to the seventies.[82] Improved techniques for matching donors and donees have vastly increased the success of unrelated donor transplants.[83] As a result, about a third of all person-to-person stem cell transplants performed worldwide in 2002 used stem cells from unrelated donors, up from almost none only a decade ago.[84] Furthermore, nearly half of all allografts worldwide now use stem cells harvested from peripheral blood rather than from bone marrow.[85] As a result of these various advances, mortality rates have also dropped for allograft recipients.

Despite these advances, SCT remains risky. Sometimes, the procedure simply does not work.[86] The most common causes of death among transplant recipients are relapse and infection.[87] Graft-versus-host disease, moderate to severe, affects 30 to 60 percent of recipients and accounts for 15 percent of all deaths after transplantation.[88] Overall, mortality is an estimated 5 to 20 percent for autologous transplants, 20 to 30 percent for allogenic sibling transplants, and up to 45 percent for transplants between unrelated individuals.[89]

Not all uses of SCT have lived up to expectations. In the mid 1990s, for example, autografts among breast cancer patients shot up dramatically in the United States and Europe without good evidence that the procedure did any good. Eventually, clinical trials showed that transplantation was no better than conventional chemotherapy for breast cancer, and transplant rates among this group declined.[90]

Number of Patients and Cost

The number of stem cell transplantations has risen explosively from approximately 10,000 worldwide in 1990 to an estimated 59,000 by

1997.[91] This increase reflects the development of autologous procedures, a greater availability of donors, better techniques for determining donor match, and greater ease of stem cell collection.[92]

Two decades ago, the British performed BMT at a rate slightly higher than in the United States. During the period from 1989 to 1991, treatment rates were virtually identical. The most recent available data suggest that stem cell transplants are now provided nearly one-third more frequently in the United States than in the United Kingdom.[93]

The per patient cost of SCT has risen sharply in both the United States and the United Kingdom. In 2001 charges in the United States ranged from $94,847 for a simple autograft to $332,742 for an umbilical cord stem cell transplant. The corresponding costs for adults in the United Kingdom were roughly one-third as large, ranging from $33,412 for a peripheral blood stem cell transplant to more than $74,000 for some allografts.[94]

Total expenditures have also skyrocketed over the past two decades. In 1981 the outlay for bone marrow transplants was about $30 million in the United States and $5 million in Britain.[95] On a population-corrected basis, the British spent two-thirds as much as Americans. By 1992 the U.S. national bill increased thirtyfold to an estimated $810 million and, by 2001, to an estimated $1.9 billion.[96] British spending for stem cell transplants in 2002 was approximately $115 million.[97] These data suggest that the British now spend less than a third as much for SCT as Americans do, adjusted for population, compared to two-thirds of relative spending a generation ago.

Despite high unit cost and tight budgets, the rate of use in Britain two decades ago was at least as high as in the United States. The most recent available data suggest that stem cell transplants are now provided relatively more often in the United States than in the United Kingdom.[98] The evolution of this therapy and the spread of its use exemplify how medical knowledge gradually accumulates and new applications are discovered. In contrast to hemophilia, a rare disease for which a single form of treatment—factor replacement—is demonstrably effective, SCT is an alternative or a supplement to other forms of treatment for many diverse diseases that, collectively, are far more common. Thus the financial stakes in making SCT freely available have become far higher than in the case of factor replacement, and the indications for use are not so clear cut.

Intensive Care

Many diagnostic and therapeutic procedures that once required hospitalization are now provided on an outpatient basis. As this trend proceeds, the modern hospital is increasingly becoming an outpatient facility for most diagnostic and therapeutic procedures and an intensive care facility for the most seriously ill. Intensive care beds account for 10 percent of all U.S. hospital beds and between 20 and 25 percent of total hospital spending—roughly $100 billion in 2002. Their role is even larger than these numbers suggest because many patients are moved to regular beds to complete recovery only after having spent some time in an intensive care unit (ICU) bed. The British devote a much smaller share of a much smaller health budget to intensive care. As a result, access to intensive care beds is far more restricted in Britain than in the United States. The paucity of such beds means that some surgery must be delayed.

What Is Intensive Care?

Intensive care did not exist formally before World War II. In embryonic form, it appeared first as the postoperative recovery room.[99] The first units specially equipped to care for the critically ill appeared in Britain in the 1960s. Not until the 1990s did most British acute care hospitals have at least one intensive care unit.[100]

Intensive care units are distinguished by intensive round-the-clock nursing, often on a one-to-one basis, with a wide range of support and equipment, notably with the capacity to provide artificial ventilation to patients, blood support, and heart rhythm control.[101] Typical intensive care units have four to fifteen beds. The smaller number is a lower bound for efficient use of costly equipment.[102] Units with more than fifteen beds are reported to present management difficulties. British ICUs typically have four to six beds and are smaller than the eight- to twelve-bed units common in the United States and most other European nations, but size varies widely within each nation.[103] U.S. hospitals may have several such units, reflecting a trend to specialize ICUs—in trauma, cardiac problems, neurological conditions, and so on.

Staffing

The British have higher standards for staffing—seven nurses per ICU bed—than do the United States and several surveyed European nations.

But they do not consistently meet their own standards; the actual average is 4.2.[104] Whether this staffing level is as good as it seems is less clear. The ratio of ICU beds to all hospital beds is so much lower in Great Britain than in the United States—2 percent versus 10 percent—that the average occupant of a British ICU bed is bound to be considerably sicker than the average ICU patient in the U.S., and more nurses may substitute for less equipment.[105]

Cost

ICUs are expensive—just how costly is subject to inescapable uncertainty. Part of the problem is one of cost accounting—the inevitable arbitrariness of deciding how much of the cost of shared facilities should be assigned to ICUs and how much to other services. Part of the problem is that most U.S. data refer not to cost but to charges, which are somewhat arbitrary and frequently negotiated. Many analysts, following a pioneering study by Louise Russell in 1979, posit that an ICU day costs three times as much as a non-ICU day, although some studies report that ICU beds generate far higher costs.[106]

Data on intensive care costs are even scarcer for the United Kingdom than for the United States. A recent study put the cost for intensive care services in the United Kingdom at approximately £700 million in 1998. If growth in bed numbers and unit costs projected in that study were realized, ICUs would have accounted for 3.4 percent of U.K. hospital spending in 2002, less than one-fifth the U.S. share.[107] To have equaled U.S. intensive care levels would have required the NHS to quintuple its spending on intensive care.

Implications

Two decades ago the gap between the U.S. and U.K. endowment of intensive care was proportionately as large but smaller absolutely. At that time, British physicians acknowledged that they could use more intensive care beds to medical advantage. But planners and physicians alike perceived the overall cost to be out of proportion, given other needs. To reach parity with the United States in the early 1980s, Britain would have had to increase its total health care budget some 10 percent. One director of an intensive care unit in a teaching hospital said,

> Such a move would be inappropriate given the enormous negative impact on other services that would have funds withdrawn from

them. This [our unit] is about right and appropriate. It balances with the rest of what goes on around here. It would be crazy [to have more beds], you see, because it would be out of proportion to what we offer in the renal unit and what we offer anywhere else.[108]

In the early 1980s, British physicians discontinued aggressive therapy for the terminally ill earlier than their American counterparts did and said they would do so even if their resources were not constrained. This claim undoubtedly reflected cultural traditions and ethical views. On the other hand, the limitation on intensive care beds and other constraints forced British physicians to practice triage. They could not routinely place a seventy-five-year-old patient with advanced metastatic cancer in an intensive care unit without realizing that they might thereby deny urgent care to a twenty-five-year-old accident victim whose life was in jeopardy. In responding to a question about whether he thought more beds in his hospital should be devoted to intensive care, a doctor in charge of an intensive care unit at one of London's leading teaching hospitals replied, "No, everybody would get bored stiff and the place would be half empty. It would be a great big sham. . . . It has to be appropriate to the surroundings."[109]

The paucity of intensive care beds still poses an obstacle to therapy. Nephrologists have complained that a lack of intensive care beds restricts kidney donations from living donors.[110] And two cardiologists said that coronary surgery is sometimes constrained by a lack of intensive care beds. Particularly during the winter, coronary and other "nonemergency" surgery sometimes has had to be deferred because acutely ill patients filled the ICU beds required for care of patients after highly invasive surgery. Some surgeons tell patients that a lack of ICU beds, real or contrived, explains why they have to wait for surgery—unless, that is, they are willing to go into private beds. Thus the scarcity of ICU facilities continues to force genuine and anguished trade-offs. But eliminating that shortage would require the sacrifice of many other services or greatly increased spending.

Summary

Even when survival is involved, resource limits force trade-offs. As technology evolves and the severity of budget limits intensifies or relaxes, these trade-offs change. As time passes, what were once new technologies become familiar and established. But when the costs are very high, as in the case of dialysis or intensive care, rationing appears to be severe and persistent. When the costs are modest, as with treatment of hemophilia and stem cell transplantation, the limits on care can be hard to detect or nonexistent. Chapter 7 examines additional considerations that influence these trade-offs. Before then, however, chapters 4 and 5 present information on the effects of resource limits when relief of pain, quality of life, or medical information is at stake.

CHAPTER FOUR

Quality of Life

Tight budgets, one might think, would more severely limit care that "merely" improves the quality of life than care that saves lives. The story is a good deal more complicated, however. Discomfort may be acute, unremitting, and disabling, or it may be merely annoying and inconvenient. The benefits of surgery providing artificial hips that return bedridden and pain-racked invalids to pain-free mobility are at least as great as the gain from briefly extending the life of terminally ill, semicomatose patients. Furthermore, replacing arthritic hips may cost less than custodial care required for patients immobilized by arthritis of the hip. In contrast, care for chronic conditions that cause protracted but not crippling discomfort, such as hernias or varicose veins, may be regarded as dispensable. Many people with chest pain from coronary disease, for example, can continue working if they take appropriate medications and avoid stress and strain.

Treatments for painful diseases that are not disabling or likely to cause imminent death would seem to be ripe candidates for rationing in a budget-constrained system. Thus one might expect the British to curtail costly surgical treatment of coronary artery disease more than hip surgery. Such, indeed, is the case. People with life-threatening diseases either receive treatment or die. Those with chronic diseases live on whether treated or not. That patients and providers respond differently to limited resources in the two cases is hardly surprising. In particular, the chronically ill may well seek care from providers outside the budget limits and pay for it themselves if resource limits necessitate denial of some care.

Hip Replacement

A frequently repeated quip about the National Health Service goes: "You wait to avoid paying or pay to avoid waiting."[1] For decades the "poster child" invoked by critics of the NHS, both at home and abroad, has been that of the hobbled patient waiting months or years for a hip replacement.

In the late 1970s, queues were long and getting longer.[2] Patients routinely waited an average of thirteen to fourteen months for hip replacements. Extreme delays ran up to five years. A quarter of a century later, queues contain even more people awaiting orthopedic surgery of all kinds—159,489 in the third quarter of fiscal year 2003–04 versus 100,105 in 1977—but the average waiting times *of those treated* has shortened. (Although "waiting lists" and "waiting times" may seem straightforward concepts, they are not. See boxed text.) In 2002 average waiting times for hip replacements in England ranged from seven to slightly under nine months, depending on the extensiveness of required surgery and methods used.[3] The Blair government subsequently tried strenuously to eliminate extremely lengthy waits and succeeded to a remarkable extent. Only two patients treated in all of England in the third quarter of 2003–04 had waited more than two years for any form of treatment. That even two patients waited so long may seem shocking, but it was a dramatic improvement over the past. The average waiting time for treated orthopedic patients was down to approximately four months.

The Procedure

Because badly deteriorated hips are both painful and disabling, doctors long sought effective ways to treat them. The most radical approach involves replacing the joint completely. The hip joint is relatively simple: a ball at the end of the femur and a socket in the pelvis. Although the hip joint is uncomplicated, devising a satisfactory prosthesis proved extremely difficult because an artificial joint must pass several demanding tests. It must be strong—most of the body's weight rests on it. It has to be durable—wear can cause serious problems and necessitate repeat surgery. It must resist corrosion by body fluids. It cannot cause inflammation. And, it must be attached securely to the femur and pelvis so that it usually does not loosen.

Waiting List Statistics

The meaning of waiting list statistics depends on at least three distinct considerations. How long does it take to get on the list? How long does it take to get off? Who is counted—those on the list at a point in time, or those who have completed their stay on the list?

NHS patients must often wait to see a consultant. Then they may have to wait to be placed on a list for hospital admission. Once on that list, they may have to wait for admission. The patient cares about total time elapsed from onset of disease to final treatment—or, as sometimes occurs, death.

Data on time spent on waiting lists are hard to interpret. One may measure how long those now on the waiting list have been on it. Or one can measure how long those treated during a given period waited. The first approach disregards the waits of those who have been treated during the period. The second disregards the waits of those who have *not* been treated. Both views are incomplete.

Furthermore, each measure is sensitive to the health authority's policy for deciding who gets treated first. In actual practice, this decision depends in some fashion on the severity of the patients' illnesses—those wounded in the London tube bombing were treated before cases awaiting prostheses to replace arthritic knees—and how long they have already waited. At one extreme, new patients might always be treated first. If the number of new cases exceeds capacity, patients not treated at first would never be treated. At the other extreme, patients who have been waiting longest might be treated next.

For any given patient flow and treatment capacity, these two approaches lead to quite different waiting list statistics. For example, suppose that 100 patients qualify for treatment at the start of each period (say, a calendar quarter), but only 80 can be treated. At the end of twelve periods—that is, after three years—960 patients would have been treated and 240 patients would be on the waiting list. But the average time spent on the waiting list by those who were treated and by those still on the list would differ sharply, depending on which treatment rule was in effect, as the table below shows:

Effect of Treatment Policy on Duration of Wait,
Twelve-Period (-Quarter) Time Span
In periods (quarters)

	Average wait	
Treatment policy	Those treated	Those still on list
A. Most recent first	0	6
B. Longest waiters first	1.1875	1.75

In this example, the choice of admissions policy B would increase the average duration of wait from nil to approximately 3.5 months for those treated and decrease the duration of wait from 1.5 years to a bit over five months for those still awaiting care.

This example involves extreme and unrealistic rules. Neither policy represents actual practice. For this reason, the example exaggerates the effects of plausible variations in admission policies. On the other hand, truncating the calculation at twelve periods (three years) understates the effects of policy choice. The implication is clear, however: changing admission policies can significantly alter a politically sensitive statistic.

The first hip replacement was done in 1923 but quickly failed. Success came only in 1962 when Sir John Charnley, an English surgeon working in a small countryside hospital, used a new polymer plastic cement developed in Britain, polymethylmethacrylate, that was tough and durable enough to hold the hip prosthesis in place. The prosthesis consisted of a plastic cup placed in the pelvis and a steel ball attached to the femur.[4]

Subsequent research has developed new materials—superalloys and ceramics—and new methods of attachment, including porous materials into which the patient's own bone grows.[5] Total replacement is usually indicated in cases of advanced osteoarthritis. In the treatment of broken hips, a common problem among the elderly, replacing only the head and neck of the femur usually suffices. Infection is a potentially catastrophic risk that can leave the patient worse off than before. A more common problem is wear of the surface of the prosthesis, which releases implant particles that cause inflammation and bone loss around the implant.

Hip replacements are successful for both old and young patients. Young patients are more likely than elderly ones to require repeat surgery, in part because the former are more likely to outlive the prosthesis and in part because the greater activity of the young is more likely to cause the prosthesis to loosen.[6] The proportion of artificial hips that loosen enough after surgery to cause discomfort or require repeat surgery has declined— from as much as 5 percent annually two decades ago to 1 to 2 percent currently. For patients with severe hip disease, however, the relief from pain provided by successful hip replacement far outweighs the risks.

Frequency of Surgery

Data on the frequency of hip replacement in Britain and the United States are hard to interpret. Several different procedures are involved, and reporting is incomplete. The previously existing gap in the population-adjusted rates of hip replacements, total and partial combined, has closed (see appendix table A-4). Furthermore, one study indicates that the rate of surgery approximately equals the estimated incidence of new hip problems.[7]

Even a small disparity between the incidence of hip problems requiring surgery and the availability of surgery can quickly lengthen or shorten waiting lists because untreated patients do not get well and may live for years. If waiting lists contain half as many patients as undergo surgery, even a 10 percent annual shortfall would double the list in five years. Similarly, a modest addition of resources can quickly cut the list.

Since modest additional resources would seem sufficient to eliminate queues, the failure of the NHS to end the notorious and well-documented waiting lists for hip surgery is puzzling. The answer is that ensuring that additional resources are used just for hip surgery is difficult. The hospital beds, operating rooms, and hospital staff necessary to eliminate waits for hip replacements are general-purpose surgical resources that can be used for many other forms of surgery. The doctors and nurses who would have decided how to use those resources would probably have placed medical criteria ahead of eliminating a public relations embarrassment. To reduce waiting lists for hip surgery, therefore, the central authorities would have had to increase spending far more than the direct cost of the added hip surgery. The government seems now to have made just such a commitment to cutting waiting lists across the board and to raising NHS spending enough to do the job.

Private Provision

In the era of lengthy waiting lists, much hip surgery was done privately— perhaps as much as 25 percent in some parts of Britain. Doctors saw patients outside the NHS and charged patients for their services. In low-income areas, the proportion of hips replaced privately was much smaller, perhaps as low as 5 percent. Such private surgery was performed in either NHS pay beds or in private hospitals. Patients paid the surgical fee and bed charges themselves or used private insurance.

Because the surgeons perform hip surgery both within the NHS and privately on a fee-for-service basis, the existence of long waiting lists for free NHS surgery created an opportunity for NHS physicians to divert patients to their lucrative private practices. When resource limits were binding, surgeons who diverted patients to their private practices, like some old-time missionaries, "did well by doing good." Such diversion sped treatment for many, even as it fattened physician incomes. The more dismaying fact was that some physicians used shortages to maneuver patients into seeing them privately. They told patients that free NHS hip surgery would be long delayed but that private care could be had quickly—for a price. Hip surgery is time consuming and exacting. Hospital stays after surgery were far lengthier in the past than they are today. Surgeons could have rationalized such diversions of cases to private practices on the grounds that several patients could be treated for other conditions in the period while a single hip surgery patient convalesced.

It is not surprising that good data on such practices have never existed. Two decades ago, a group of orthopedic surgeons in one district general hospital gained some notoriety for allegedly doing a large part of their hip surgery on a private basis.[8] Some consultant physicians acknowledged at that time that they had heard rumors that such practices occurred, but most denied that they or any of their colleagues engaged in them. The very possibility of waiting-list manipulation is one reason why some members of the Labour party long opposed allowing NHS physicians to practice privately part time.

And yet, from a broader standpoint, channeling patients into the private sector may serve NHS interests. Patients who pay for their own treatment free up resources in a budget-constrained system that can be used to care for others. Few would condone actions that drove the acutely ill or the poor to seek care privately. But the decision to ration means that some beneficial care will be denied that would be available in an unconstrained system. In that event, focusing limited resources on illnesses that cannot wait and patients who cannot pay serves the general interest. In fact, official reports have endorsed the practice of using private care to shorten waiting times.[9]

Coronary Revascularization

Coronary artery disease is the most frequent cause of death in both the United States and Great Britain. Most commonly, arteries that supply blood to the heart become partially or completely blocked. When the blockage is nearly complete, patients may suffer angina pectoris—Latin for "strangling in the chest." The pain, often severe, commonly radiates to the left arm and upward to the neck or jaw. The pain results from partial blockage of coronary arteries or spasm of coronary arteries which restricts blood flow, starving the heart muscle for oxygen.[10] Blockages can result from either blood clots or the buildup of fatty deposits called plaque. Complete blockage causes a heart attack. The portion of the heart that is denied oxygen dies unless the blockage is quickly cleared.[11]

Physicians have understood these processes for nearly 200 years. Until recently, however, they could do little to prevent the disease or treat the results. For angina they could provide only brief symptomatic relief with nitroglycerin and related drugs. For victims of heart attacks, they could prescribe little other than bed rest. The drug digitalis was believed to ease discomfort of victims of congestive heart failure, a condition that may result when the heart muscle weakens or is partly destroyed by a coronary.

In recent years, the menu of treatments for angina, coronary blockages, and heart failure has grown enormously. Dozens of new drugs can improve function in the failing heart, reduce or even reverse the buildup of plaque and the likelihood of clots that will cause heart attacks, and prevent or reduce permanent damage when heart attacks strike. Many of the treatments do not demonstrably extend life but do improve its quality. Statins, first marketed in 1987, reduce serum cholesterol, a blood constituent associated with the progress of coronary artery disease.[12] Two surgical interventions—coronary artery bypass surgery (CABG, often pronounced "cabbage") and percutaneous transluminal coronary angioplasty ("angioplasty," for short)—have come into common use. In 2002 approximately 1.7 million patients in the United States and 82,000 in the United Kingdom underwent CABG or angioplasty.[13] Most angioplasty procedures now include the use of stents, metal mesh cylinders that can be expanded by using a balloon to sustain an opening in an artery. Most stents now used in the United States and some in Britain are coated with anticlotting drugs to discourage future plaque buildups. The need for CABG and angioplasty would be even greater than it is were it not for the large menu of new drugs that slow the progress and relieve the symptoms of coronary disease and break up blood clots that cause the complete blockages resulting in death of part of the heart muscle.

Method of Treatment

In recent decades surgical procedures have been developed for improving the flow of blood to the heart. Coronary artery bypass surgery was first performed in 1962.[14] This procedure became possible only after the development of a machine that routes the patient's blood flow away from the heart, removes carbon dioxide from the blood, reoxygenates it, and returns it to the circulation.[15] With the help of this "heart-lung" machine, the heart can be stopped from pumping long enough to permit surgery on the heart itself.

CABG is the preferred therapy for patients with blockages that angioplasty cannot open (such as those at branching points in coronary arteries), with very extensive coronary disease, or who suffer heart attacks during angioplasty. Either angioplasty or coronary surgery is clearly indicated in patients with disabling chest pain that is unresponsive to drugs and behavioral changes. These interventions also help patients with "silent" ischemia, a shortage of blood flow to the heart that causes no pain but can interfere with the heart's pumping, causing fainting or death. For the roughly 10 percent of patients in whom the left main coronary artery is narrowed by more than 50 percent, surgery not only relieves pain more than drugs do but also results in improved survival.[16] When three or more arteries are affected—about 30 percent of all cases—or if the left anterior descending artery is involved with diminished function of the left ventricle, there is also some evidence that surgery prolongs life as well as reduces pain.

Coronary artery surgery initially was extremely invasive and very risky. The operation is performed only after the cardiologist or radiologist makes an angiogram, a detailed x-ray of the heart. Increasingly, disease is detected among asymptomatic patients through stress tests and scans. A tube is inserted into an artery, and a radiopaque dye is injected to make the coronary blood vessels visible and pinpoint the number and extent of blockages. In ordinary CABG the surgeon saws open the patient's sternum to gain access to the heart. The surgeon then stops the heart, removes a blood vessel from the patient's leg or chest, and uses it to reroute blood circulation to bypass the blocked section of the coronary artery. For some blockages on the heart's surface, surgeons can now sometimes avoid the need to split the sternum and use the heart-lung machine by making a small incision in the chest and operating on the beating heart. The mortality rate from surgery averages 2.4 percent but is as little as 0.5 percent if the procedure is performed by an experienced surgeon in a facility that does such procedures often.[17]

Angioplasty is an offshoot of angiography. It was invented by a Swiss physician, Andreas R. Gruentzig, and first performed in 1977 in San Francisco. A catheter with a small balloon just behind the tip is typically inserted through a small incision, usually in the groin, and threaded upward into the narrowed coronary artery. At that point the physician inflates the balloon, with the goal of expanding the obstructive lesion and thereby enlarging the arterial opening. When successful, the procedure increases blood flow through the previously partly blocked artery, relieving pain and improving heart function. If the blockage is particularly hard, the physician may use a laser or a small drill, attached to the end of the catheter. Once the artery has been opened, the catheter is withdrawn, the small incision is closed, and the patient can usually go home the same or next day. Occasionally, complete blockage occurs during angioplasty, and the patient immediately undergoes coronary bypass surgery. Angioplasty is performed about twice as often as bypass surgery in the United States because it avoids the surgical trauma associated with CABG and recovery typically is quick.

Unfortunately, many early angioplasties provided only temporary relief because blockages soon reappeared in recently opened arteries. To prevent such "restenosis," physicians began to insert small metal mesh sleeves, or stents, after the arterial passage was widened. These stents are expanded against the arterial wall with the balloon and are left in place when the balloon is removed. Stents improved outcomes, but in about 20–30 percent of cases, the mesh sleeves became sites for scar tissue, new deposits, or blood clots, and blockages recurred within a year. To reduce this problem, stents now are usually coated with drugs that dissolve gradually and retard tissue buildup. Such "drug-eluting" stents reduce by 60 to 70 percent the probability of blockage during the nine months after the procedure.[18] Their use has become routine in the United States.

Cost

Both CABG and angioplasty require advanced medical equipment and highly skilled physicians, nurses, and technicians. Accordingly, they are expensive: in the United States in 2002, CABGs cost an estimated $60,853 per patient, and angioplasties cost $33,077 for percutaneous procedures (including costs for the procedures and physicians' charges). In 2002, 515,000 CABGs and 1.2 million angioplasties were performed. As a result, total outlays for these procedures were *very* large—nearly $74 billion, or about 5 percent of total health care spending, and about 8 percent of U.S. spending on direct patient care, five times the share in 1982.[19]

Though costs were staggeringly large in 2002, they are almost certainly higher now and headed up—probably *way* up—for three reasons. The first is the advent of drug-eluting stents. Their use has spread steadily since 2002. Drug-coated stents cost about $3,000 each, three times the cost of the bare stents they replaced. Nearly two stents per angioplasty, on average, are used. By the end of 2003, drug-eluting stents were used in an estimated three-fourths of all angioplasties.

The second cost-increasing force is research showing that angioplasty generally improves outcomes for victims of heart attacks. The cost of the previously preferred treatment—administration of drugs that speed dissolution of artery-blocking clots—is far lower. Studies in the early 1990s documented that providing angioplasty after coronary occlusions improved outcomes but that patients should not be moved to another facility if the hospital to which they were initially admitted lacked the capacity to perform angioplasties. Later studies showed that even those patients who are moved benefit from the procedure if it is performed soon enough.[20] Many hospitals that lack the capacity to perform angioplasties are near facilities that do. Accordingly, the number of heart attack victims receiving angioplasties is bound to increase.

The third force driving up spending is demography. The leading edge of the baby boom generation has reached the age when the incidence of heart attacks is high. As more individuals age into these disease-prone years, a growing population—multiplied by an increased rate of treatment within that population and compounded by increasingly costly treatment methods—portends very rapid increases in spending.

Relative Frequency of Treatment in the United States and the United Kingdom

The gap in treatment rates between the United States and the United Kingdom has been huge for more than two decades. In the late 1970s, the annual CABG surgery rate was 490 per million in the United States (1979) and 55 per million in the United Kingdom (1977).[21] The U.S. CABG rate was about three times the angioplasty rate. The United Kingdom did not report data on angioplasties, presumably because so few were performed that it was not worth counting them. At that time, the U.S. revascularization rate was at least ten times that in the United Kingdom.

The incidence of both procedures has grown enormously. By 2002 the combined CABG and angioplasty rate in the United States had increased more than twelvefold to an annual rate of 5,967 per million. In the United Kingdom, the combined angioplasty–CABG rate reached 1,380 per million. Though a twenty-five-fold increase over 1977 and more than twice the U.S. rate in that year, the 2002 U.K. rate remained only one-fourth of the contemporary U.S. rate, and the absolute gap had widened.[22]

Qualitative, as well as quantitative, differences are striking. In 1996, 11 percent of U.S. patients received angioplasty within one day of a heart attack. Two years later, by which time the rate had doubtless risen in the United States, the proportion of patients similarly treated in Scotland was only 4 percent. The British speedily adopted bare metal stents as standard in angioplasties—nearly 90 percent of angioplasties performed in 2001 in the United Kingdom used stents.[23] On the other hand, the British have shunned the newer drug-coated stents, while their use has become routine in the United States. Various studies indicate that angioplasty and drug-coated stents improve patients' outcomes. If one takes such quality improvement into account, these technologies may even have reduced the price of treatment for heart disease as well as increased the likelihood of desirable medical outcomes, even as they have increased total spending.[24]

Mortality from Heart Disease

Mortality from heart disease has dropped strikingly over the last generation in the United States, the United Kingdom, and most other nations. The countries of Eastern Europe and former members of the Soviet Union are notable exceptions. The pace and timing of improvement in the United States and Britain have differed, however.[25] In 1968 the age-adjusted mortality rate from heart disease was 25 percent lower in the United Kingdom than in the United States. By 2000 the U.K. rate was 7 percent higher.

In the mid-twentieth century, U.S. mortality from coronary disease was among the highest in the world. From 1968 through 1976, faster emergency response times and improved cardiac techniques contributed to declining coronary disease mortality.[26] For reasons that are unclear, mortality from coronary disease increased in Great Britain during this period. Perhaps the British population suffered long-delayed effects of wartime hardships endured years before. Perhaps an unhealthful diet, smoking, and other factors were at work. Throughout the 1970s, coronary disease and stroke mortality declined in the United States, probably because of the growing use of diuretics and the introduction of beta-blockers to control hypertension.[27] Over the succeeding two decades, the drop in coronary disease mortality continued in the United States. Improvements greatly exceeded those in the United Kingdom. Starting in the late 1980s, however, mortality rates from coronary disease began to fall faster in the United Kingdom than in the United States, despite the far higher U.S. use of advanced medical therapies.

Estimates indicate that medical interventions accounted for much of the decline in coronary disease mortality in the United States between 1975 and 1995. These interventions included low-tech approaches, such as prescribing aspirin at the onset of or soon after a heart attack, and newer clot-busting drugs. They also included highly sophisticated surgical procedures.[28] In addition, environmental conditions and diet improved. Tobacco consumption began to decline. Routine screening for hypertension, an important risk factor for both heart disease and stroke, became common in the United States, as did widespread use of various drugs to control hypertension.[29] Similar routine screening was, and remains, uncommon in Great Britain. As one cardiologist put it:

> By and large, people in this country would not, if they were perfectly fit and well, go and have things like their cholesterol done. . . . We don't have annual physicals in this country, or biennially or however frequently it's done. . . . You go to the doctor when you're ill. . . . The only national screening program here is the breast cancer screening, which is done at three-year intervals on women between age fifty and sixty-five. [Note: The American Cancer Society recommends annual mammograms for all women over the age of forty.[30]] . . . But when you're talking about an aging population, there is no national screening that goes on, no.

British officials at a meeting to develop local prescribing guidelines for statins concluded that prescribing them for primary prevention—to forestall the development of the first signs of disease—in low-risk patients was not worth the investment. ("I mean these people aren't in pain. The statins won't make them feel better or anything.") Many U.S. cardiologists would probably agree, but they set a stricter standard than do their British counterparts for distinguishing between high- and low-risk patients. The British classify as high risk a patient judged to have a 30 percent likelihood of experiencing a serious cardiac event in the next ten years. The U.S. standard for treatment is a 20 percent risk and extends indications for treatment to include a family history of heart disease, a criterion not mentioned in British guidelines.[31]

Explanations for Treatment Differences

Four possible explanations might account for the very large difference in treatment rates between the United States and the United Kingdom: differences in epidemiology and aggressiveness of treatment, in physician and patient attitudes, in resources, and in the way physicians are paid.

EPIDEMIOLOGY. The relative frequency of coronary disease in the two countries, detected and undetected, is, by definition, unknown. Nor can simple trends in mortality resolve how much differences in treatment contributed to the fall in coronary mortality in both nations or whether they were or were not the dominant factor. The likelihood of detection is higher in the United States because of more frequent routine physical examinations. Thus it is unclear whether underlying disease is more or less common, despite lower mortality from heart disease in the United States than in the United Kingdom.

What is clear is that, once detected, coronary disease has been and is treated far more aggressively in the United States than in Great Britain. Furthermore, medical targets, such as better control of blood pressure, serum cholesterol, and other conditions associated with an increased risk of developing or dying from coronary disease, are also more ambitious in the United States than in Great Britain. And research is continuing to suggest clinical gains from meeting lower and lower thresholds.[32]

ATTITUDES. By common perception, resource limits and differences in attitudes toward medical care interact. The British spend less on health care in part because, on the average, physicians believe that conservative medicine is the best medicine and in part because patients in Britain are less demanding than those in the United States. These attitudes have clearly been conditioned by, and are a way of accommodating to, decades of tight budgets that flatly exclude approaches to medical care that U.S. patients and physicians alike take for granted.

Twenty years ago, British physicians relied on medical treatment—specifically, drugs to ease cardiac burden and changes in diet and lifestyle—until coronary disease had advanced well beyond the point at which U.S. physicians would have prescribed surgery. Soon after two calcium channel blockers, nifedipine and verapamil, were introduced in Great Britain—and well before they had been approved for use in the United States—one British consulting cardiologist said that such drugs "appreciably raised the threshold at which patients were referred for surgical treatment."[33] About the same time, however, another distinguished cardiologist expressed doubt that differences in drug therapy accounted for the difference in coronary surgery in the two countries. The medical indications for surgery were similar in the United States and Britain. However, in determining when that threshold has been reached, British and U.S. experts have long differed strikingly. In 1982, when revascularization was about ten times as common in the United States as in Great Britain, a *Lancet* editorial took a "go slow" attitude, declaring that coronary artery surgery should be used only in the presence of "disabling chest pain, when full medical therapy has failed."[34] At almost the same time, a report in the *New England Journal of Medicine* summarized the view that surgery should be based not only on whether it would improve life expectancy but also "on . . . the patient's priorities."[35] An article in

Science on the consensus on coronary artery surgery in the early 1980s reported that "many patients demand surgery rather than medical treatment" and quoted a physician that "male patients often 'want to be seen as men, as husbands, as providers, and they are willing to risk their lives at the time of the operation so as not to change their life styles.'"[36]

British medical journals have long recognized that more coronary artery surgery and angioplasty should be done in Britain and that, as one cardiologist put it, "more CABG surgery would be carried out if the capacity for it increased significantly." But another cardiologist noted that even "in . . . areas [where] there is in practice no limitation on resources . . . the rate of CABG surgery is lower than in the U.S."

That two decades and a huge increase in treatment in both countries have not erased these differences became clear in several recent conversations with British cardiologists and foreign physicians with clinical experience in Great Britain. Even in 2004, one cardiologist stated that "in this country . . . we have a tradition in the health service that you don't offer the treatment until it's absolutely necessary." Another British cardiologist with clinical experience in both the United States and Great Britain reported:

> Over here, simply because of the logistics and limited resources, many times the patient will be watched. If the pain doesn't persist and there doesn't seem to be any urgency, one will discharge the patient, do an exercise test, make sure that there are no ECG [electrocardiogram] changes when the heart is stressed and bring the patient back later. And so, one is doing less of that procedure than one would be doing almost automatically in the USA.

That patients acquiesce in such parsimonious treatment surprises even British physicians. According to a South Yorkshire general practitioner, commenting in 1995 with apparent admiration, "People from round here cope. They don't like making a fuss. They have a depth of character." And a colleague added, "Patients will be getting angina on a daily basis and . . . they brush it off. It's almost par for the course. I'm astonished at the laid-backness about this."[37] Finally, a U.S. cardiologist with extensive experience in the United Kingdom said,

> My impression is that in general in the United Kingdom, there are much more rigid criteria to institute life-saving procedures. . . . I saw that over and over. Where certain procedures would just not be

offered because it was not felt appropriate because these people were elderly. And they were going to die anyway. . . . I don't think it is a capacity issue. I think it is a philosophical issue. I think philosophically they're much more willing to accept death in the elderly without major intervention, more so than in the United States.

RESOURCES AND METHODS OF PAYMENT. While differences in national character doubtlessly exist, biology has not identified a gene coding for stiff upper lips. Stoical attitudes emerge in part to cope with inescapable medical constraints imposed by harsh fiscal reality.

The issue of physical capacity arose repeatedly in recent conversations. A British cardiologist who was fully aware of research documenting the benefits of angioplasty after heart attacks explained, "I've got a waiting list for angioplasty for six months from my elective work. . . . We would like to go to acute infarct angioplasty, but . . . there are very few centers in the United Kingdom doing that." A European cardiologist with British experience reported the case of a patient who crossed the English Channel for treatment after learning that he required coronary surgery in three arteries. Despite the diagnosis, the patient's surgeon told him that the operating room schedule was so tight that there would be time to operate on only one artery. Two cardiologists reported that coronary surgery is sometimes constrained by a lack of intensive care beds.

A lack of capacity—a paucity of centers with resources to provide advanced care and of cardiologists—severely limits the intensity of coronary care. There are 53 percent more cardiologists in New Jersey, which has about one-seventh of the United Kingdom's population, than in all of the United Kingdom.[38] Most British patients with angina are therefore treated by primary care physicians who are not trained to perform or prescribe angiograms and may not be fully versed in the latest research on management of coronary disease. A majority of general practitioners around Southampton reported that they refer only one-fourth of their patients with stable angina to a hospital physician and one-tenth or fewer to a regional center. These rates are consistent with national estimates.[39]

Official British medical guidance justifies neither the low referral rates to secondary care nor limited use of angiograms thereafter. The Royal College of Physicians and the British Cardiac Society declared that *suspected* angina is reason enough to refer patients for further investigation because it is difficult to gauge the seriousness of coronary disease by the severity of a patient's symptoms, particularly because the medical risk of referral is nil.[40] Nonetheless, in 1998 only an estimated 33 percent of patients with stable angina were referred to secondary care by their GPs. Even more striking is the fact that only 69 percent of patients with myocardial infarction were referred for secondary care.[41]

One U.S. physician who had practiced in a part of Great Britain where coronary mortality is particularly high described the consequences of inadequate resources:

> What I saw happening I found very disturbing. If the waiting lists are long [for coronary surgery], you just sort of don't do as many. What I saw happening is that in Great Britain, where smoking is fairly prevalent, diet is not exactly low in fat or carbohydrates, there was a significant amount of vascular and coronary disease. You see people at a relatively young age, in their early to mid-fifties, productive, working, but developing angina to the extent that their angina was severe enough that they actually got studied. And often, we would find three-vessel coronary disease, and they would then be referred for a coronary bypass. But the individuals would be incapacitated by the angina. They would go on a waiting list. And on the waiting lists, about 20 percent of them died of coronaries before they got a bypass.

The large differences in rates of coronary surgery and angioplasty should be set against the decades-long persistence of much lower rates of surgery of all kinds in Britain as compared to the United States.[42] The difference between the systems used to pay surgeons and hospitals in the United States and Great Britain is frequently cited as a possible reason for different surgical rates. Fee-for-service payment is typical in the United States.[43] Most British specialists and the minority of U.S. surgeons employed by health maintenance organizations are salaried employees. Rates of surgery on patients enrolled in U.S. HMOs are lower than overall surgery rates. Physicians paid on a fee-for-service basis have a stronger incentive to perform surgery of all kinds than do physicians paid on salary.[44] As one American cardiologist put it: "The entrepreneurial aspect of surgery in this country makes it imperative for surgeons to pursue the recruitment of patients aggressively. There is not only the major income motivation, but also the need to meet all sorts of state standards in terms of the number of cases done per year, solely to justify a cardiac surgical unit's existence (greater than 250 a year in many states)."

Unsurprisingly, British consultants are not immune to such incentives.

Problem: Manipulation of Waiting Lists

Reports of waiting list manipulation involve cardiologists as well as orthopedic surgeons. When doing an angiogram, U.S. cardiologists like to perform any indicated angioplasties while the patient is sedated. This practice avoids the admittedly minor risk from introducing the catheter twice, once to identify lesions and a second time to widen the narrowed artery. Some British cardiologists reportedly wait until patients awake after the angioplasty, inform them of any arterial narrowing, and tell them that they must wait some time for a free angioplasty through the National Health Service. But, the patient is told, an angioplasty is available without delay if the patient is willing to see the cardiologist privately for a fee. The patient cited earlier, who crossed the English Channel for coronary surgery, had been informed by his surgeon that he could have surgery for all three of his partly occluded arteries if the patient agreed to surgery in a private hospital. The reason the patient rejected this option revealed the continuing importance of NHS hospitals in providing comprehensive services not available in many private facilities. The patient had previously received a kidney transplant. The private hospital lacked dialysis facilities, which would be life saving if the patient's kidney graft failed during coronary surgery.

Private practice can be particularly lucrative in the United Kingdom. It is entirely unregulated, and physicians can charge whatever the market will bear. Some fees reportedly vastly exceed those in the United States. In the past, consultants could elect a contract that excluded private practice or one that paid them one-eleventh less on the basis that they worked eleven half days a week and would take one for private practice. In actuality, consultants were expected to work five full days for the NHS and could spend as much of the rest of their time as they wished in private practice. Some consultants reportedly delegated much of their NHS work to lower-ranking physicians—registrars and senior registrars. Under the new contracts, which pay more than the old ones did, the content of NHS work is defined, and the scope of private practice is defined and must not interfere with NHS work.[45]

What Difference Does It Make?

Evidence that advanced medical therapy has contributed to the decline in mortality from coronary disease is powerful. Nonetheless, rates of use of these therapies are poorly correlated with mortality rates. One comparison of U.S. rates of use of these procedures with rates in Scotland, Finland, and the Canadian province of Ontario found that the United States performed two to three times as much bypass surgery and three to five times as many angioplasties as were done in these three places. The proportion of U.S. patients dying within one year after an initial heart attack was lower than that in Scotland or Finland but indistinguishable from that in Ontario.[46] This finding is consistent with the view that additional use of modern medical techniques could improve coronary mortality in Scotland. But it also supports the view of British physicians that although Britain uses advanced technology too little, the United States may be using it too much. And it is consistent with findings that U.S. physicians neglect low-cost interventions, such as prescribing aspirin and beta-blockers, that can also strongly influence mortality after heart attacks.

Conclusion

For many years British residents experienced painful delays awaiting hip replacements and other surgical procedures. Recent budget increases have dramatically reduced the average delay before hip surgery. British use of advanced technology to treat coronary disease has increased sharply over the past two decades but is still less than in the United States. Even increasing British health care budgets seems unlikely to close the gap completely. On the other hand, it may well be that the United States is using advanced technology to excess.

The many years of limited budgets seem to have fostered or reinforced attitudes among British patients and providers alike that are now partly independent of externally imposed limits. U.S. patients and physicians would likely experience similar shifts in what is regarded as appropriate care if resource limits were to foreclose the provision of all beneficial care. Similarly, the growth in funding of the NHS not only reflects the wishes of an increasingly demanding populace but may well contribute to that very assertiveness. The next chapter examines how budget limits condition the use of diagnostic procedures over which patients exercise relatively little influence.

CHAPTER FIVE

Diagnoses

Patients are sometimes comforted by the myth that physicians are inerrant, a delusion some unkind medical critics allege that physicians welcome. This belief that physicians seldom err has certain advantages: it increases patients' willingness to adhere to prescribed regimens, and it alleviates anxieties that can obstruct recovery. But as all competent doctors and well-informed patients realize, it is false. In fact, physicians are usually at least a bit unsure about the precise cause of various signs and symptoms, as well as about the best method of treatment.

Physicians acquire information in many ways. They ask questions. They perform physical examinations. They use their senses of touch and smell. And, increasingly, they prescribe various tests. Tests to measure the concentration of constituents of blood, urine, sputum, and other body components have long been available. Newer tests identify genetic markers associated with the advent of various diseases. Simple x-ray examinations, once the only noninvasive way to look inside the human body, and exploratory surgery have been supplemented or replaced by ultrasound, radioisotopes, magnetic resonance imaging, fiber optics, and computed tomography—technologies that often supply more and better information than common x-rays. But such information is costly and does not always translate into better treatment or improved patient outcomes.

An ideal test is cheap, produces no side effects, and is always right in two senses: it correctly identifies a pathology whenever it is present, and it correctly indicates its absence whenever it is not present.[1] Inaccuracy in either sense is clearly costly when a beneficial treatment is available. But signaling an abnormal condition when none is present is also damaging because it may expose healthy patients to needless worry, costly treatments, and perhaps to harmful side effects. A new test may reduce one but not both of these errors. In such cases, great care must be exercised in selecting patients on whom the test will be used, particularly when the new test is more costly or risky than the old.[2] But even accurate tests can be worthless—or worse—when, for instance, effective treatments are unavailable for the condition. For example, while a test exists to identify the gene that results in amyotrophic lateral sclerosis (Lou Gehrig's disease), possible carriers of the gene sometimes elect not to have the test as no effective treatment for the condition exists.

What would be the impact of resource limits on investments in improved diagnostic technology? Decisionmakers subject to resource limits are likely to be particularly cautious and skeptical before investing in allegedly superior diagnostic procedures, because even tests with greater accuracy may not improve diagnoses, treatments, or outcomes. Health care decisionmakers who are subject to budget limits would seek evidence that the new information justifies added costs and risks to patients from side effects.

Comparison of investments in Britain and the United States in two forms of diagnostic equipment supports those expectations. British scientists pioneered the development of computed tomography (CT) scanning. This technique noninvasively provides detailed information about body structures. Nevertheless, Britain initially bought few such scanners. Even now it has only about one-fourth as many per capita as the United States does. The adoption of the next generation of noninvasive imaging devices using magnetic resonance followed a similar pattern. Not only have the British bought fewer machines, they use them less intensively than do U.S. hospitals and radiological centers. The same pattern showed up in British use of the still newer scanning technology, positron emission tomography (PET).

The crucial question is whether these economies have seriously compromised the quality of medical care. Many health economists and planners—and some physicians—hold that the United States has overinvested in CT scanners and magnetic resonance imaging machines. Whether this allegation is correct is a particularly complicated and important question because the large and growing market for advanced imaging devices has spurred research and innovation that has improved the machines and extended their uses.

Technological advances, particularly in CT scanners, have been extremely rapid, in large measure because manufacturers saw a quickly growing market. Major improvements in the quality and capability of the machines have resulted. New uses for them in treatment, as well as diagnosis, have been discovered. It seems unlikely that the pace of advance in hardware, software, and application would have been as impressive if the market were smaller. The ultimate questions of whether and how much these advances have improved patient outcomes are even harder to answer.

CT Scanners

Until the late nineteenth century, the internal workings of the human body could be observed only through exploratory surgery. In 1895 a German physicist, Wilhelm Roentgen, discovered that x-rays passed through the human body, activated photographic film, and revealed the internal skeletal structure, a discovery for which he later received the first Nobel prize in physics. X-ray photographs readily distinguish bone and fat from other tissue. Ordinary x-rays cannot, however, differentiate among other types of soft tissue. Although noninvasive in the sense that they spare physicians the need to cut patients open to look inside them, x-ray photographs are not harmless because they require the use of ionizing radiation that marginally increases the likelihood of various cancers, can damage reproductive cells, and can cause birth defects if used on pregnant women. Although not initially recognized, these risks are now well understood.

In 1972 Godfrey Hounsfield of EMI Laboratories and Allan McLeod Cormack of Tufts University independently invented what was initially called computed axial tomography—now shortened to computed tomography. Computed tomography (CT) exploits the physical fact that different types of soft tissue, as well as bone, weaken (or attenuate) the x-rays in varying degrees. A CT image, or scan, starts with multiple x-rays taken by an x-ray tube rotating around the patient's body. Computer software then integrates these photographs into a single image or "slice." Sequential slices made by a CT scanner can distinguish normal brain tissue from brain tumor or a normal from an abscessed liver. The CT scanner makes it possible to identify the size of such abnormalities and to pinpoint their location. To improve image quality, some examinations include the administration of contrast media—substances that are opaque to x-rays. In 1979 Hounsfield and Cormack shared the Nobel prize in medicine for their discovery.

CT scanning has been marked by dramatic improvements in hardware and software and by rapid learning of new applications.[3] The scanners available in 1980 acquired images of a patient's body one slice at a time. Each scan took three minutes or longer per exposure. Computer analysis of the results took still more time. The rotating x-ray source would slow and come to a halt between each slice. Imaging was so slow that scanners could not be used effectively on the human torso because the movement of normal breathing blurred the image. For that reason, scanners initially were designed for the head only.

Today's machines are vastly faster. Four rotations of the scanner per second are now possible. A single or multiple x-ray emitter rotates continuously around the patient in a spiral fashion. Units that rotate a single x-ray tube around the patient are referred to as spiral scanners. More expensive units, which use multiple x-ray beams, are referred to as multislice scanners. A two-slice machine became available in 1992, a four-slice machine in 1998, and thirty-two-slice and forty-slice scanners in 2003. Sixty-four-slice scanners that produced images in one-third of a second—192 slices a second—became available in 2004.[4] New scanners can now be used on any part of the body, such as the lungs, during a single breath-hold of five to ten seconds.[5] Improved software enables three-dimensional images of whole organs.[6]

Medical experience and increased speed and clarity of images have opened up new applications for CT scans. As a result, radiology has split into two distinct medical fields: diagnostic and interventional radiology. Diagnostic radiologists, for example, identify the presence, size, and location of tumors. Radiation oncologists plan cancer radiotherapy and monitor the tumor's response. The images of complex fractures and facial trauma have become valuable inputs for surgeons who plan reconstructive surgery. Interventional radiologists can now guide biopsies, place some stents, and guide the ablation of cancerous tissue. In the last procedure, a needle is inserted into a tumor, which is then destroyed or reduced by radio waves. Because of improvements in imaging speed and clarity, experiments are under way to use CT scanning to replace invasive colonoscopy and angiography of coronary arteries.[7] CT scans have rendered obsolete a number of diagnostic procedures that are less accurate, create discomfort for the patient, carry significant risks, or cost more than CT scans.[8]

Cost

The quality- and inflation-adjusted price of CT scanners has plummeted since their introduction. In the early 1980s, a new top-of-the-line CT scanner cost about $700,000. It could provide one slice every five minutes. Stripped-down and reconditioned models could be had for much less, some for under $100,000.[9] By 2004 prices of consumer goods in general were roughly twice what they had been in 1980. A new top-of-the line, multislice spiral scanner that could provide 196 slices per second cost $1.2 million. Used and refurbished versions can be purchased for $150,000 to $400,000, respectively. New, single-slice scanners delivered better images faster than had single-slice machines two decades before and cost about half as much ($325,000). According to a seller of used equipment, machines similar to those used in the 1980s had become obsolete and were not available for purchase, even used.[10]

Adjusted for inflation and image quality, the cost per scan, like that of machines, has fallen sharply. Because fixed outlays account for much of the total cost of CT scans, average cost depends on the number of scans per machine as well as on the price of the machine. CT costs depend also on the part of the body scanned, whether or not contrast is injected to enhance the image, and whether or not the procedure is a diagnostic or guided surgical procedure.[11] In 1976 the estimated cost per scan in the United States ranged from about $220 if the machine was used for 2,600 scans a year to about $340 if the machine was used for 1,300 scans a year.[12] A recent study reported the cost of an unenhanced head scan at $189, while a guided biopsy was estimated to cost over $500.[13] Another study highlighted the sensitivity of average cost to volume. Cost per scan ranged from $139 if the machine was open at all hours to $208 if the machine was open only for a forty-hour work week.[14] Cost per scan in Britain is now comparable to that in the United States. According to the British Department of Health, the average procedural cost of a diagnostic CT scan in English NHS hospitals in 2001 was £119 ($172 at then-prevailing exchange rates).[15] Twenty years earlier, costs in Britain were significantly lower than in the United States.[16] The overall price level nearly doubled over this period, the number of slices per unit time increased, and image quality improved. These facts mean that the real cost of a scan fell enormously.

Number of Scanners and Scans Performed

Over the past quarter century, Britain has had fewer CT scanners per million population than the United States. The relative gap has narrowed, but the absolute gap has widened. In 1980 the United States had 6.5 CT scanners per million population, compared with 1.1 per million in the United Kingdom. By 2001 the number in the United States had risen to 29.4 per million and in the United Kingdom to 7.1 per million.[17] As of 2003, the United Kingdom had fewer scanners on a population-adjusted basis than at least five other developed countries.

Hard data on the number of scans performed are scarce. The best single estimate puts the number of scans done in the United States at 36.6 million or 128,000 per million in 2001.[18] The British Department of Health reported that 30,297 scans per million population were performed in English NHS hospitals in 2001, just under one-fourth as many as in the United States.[19] This comparison excludes any scans undertaken in private facilities in England.[20]

Two decades ago one radiologist said that any hospital with 200 or more beds and a diverse caseload could justify having a CT scanner. By this criterion, the United States eventually should have more than 3,000 scanners. A National Institutes of Health consensus panel reached a similar conclusion.[21] U.S. hospitals reached this standard in 1985. According to British radiologists, the United Kingdom had not reached this standard in 2004. Starting in 2001, the Blair government began to invest heavily in the purchase of new scanners. This program increased the stock by nearly 50 percent over the succeeding three years. So much was invested in hardware, in fact, that a lack of trained personnel to operate the machines—radiologists and radiographers (the British term for what in the United States are called "technicians")—was reported to have caused some hospitals to reject highly advanced equipment offered to them.

Magnetic Resonance Imaging

The marriage of medicine, chemistry, physics, and computer science produced a wholly different mode of imaging the internal workings of the human body—magnetic resonance imaging (MRI). MRI first entered medical practice in the early 1980s. By 2002 more than 22,000 MRI devices worldwide performed more than 60 million examinations.

The procedure was first called nuclear magnetic resonance imaging. Concerned that the word "nuclear" would spook patients frightened of dangerous radioactive substances, MRI practitioners jettisoned the "radioactive" adjective. In fact, MRI does not use ionizing radiation and is therefore safer than other imaging techniques, such as common x-ray and CT scanners.[22] MRI functions by exposing the body to a strong magnetic field that causes the nuclei of hydrogen atoms—a major constituent of water, the principal constituent of human bodies—to line up along one axis. A radio beam is then focused in a particular direction through a virtual "slice" of the body, causing a tiny fraction of these nuclei to absorb energy and change rotational direction along two axes. When the radio beam is turned off, the nuclei return to their original alignment. In the process, they emit the radio energy they have previously absorbed. Different tissues emit energy at various rates, permitting sensors to form an image of the slice. The radio beam can be aimed at different angles through the body, a feature that permits a picture in any desired orientation without requiring the patient to change position.

For the various discoveries leading up to the development of MRI, two Nobel prizes were awarded. The first, in physics, was awarded in 1952 to Felix Bloc, a Swiss-born Stanford University physicist, and Edward Purcell, an American-born Harvard professor, for their discovery of the phenomenon of nuclear magnetic resonance. The second, in physiology and medicine, was awarded in 2003 to Paul Lauterbur and Peter Mansfield for developing medically important applications for magnetic resonance imaging. Ironically, the paper by Lauterbur was initially rejected by *Nature* because referees deemed its significance too narrow for inclusion in that journal.[23]

MRI images are sometimes superior to those generated by other imaging methods. As hardware and complementary software improved and knowledge accumulated, additional uses of magnetic resonance imaging emerged. Magnetic resonance spectroscopy can identify the chemical composition of tissues. Magnetic resonance angiography is used to measure blood flow and map the anatomy of larger arteries. Functional magnetic resonance is used extensively in research on neural activity inside the brain. These technically dazzling advances leave open the central question—whether and in what situations they improve patient outcomes.

Number of Machines and Examinations

As with CT scanners, the United States has far more MRI machines than do the British—4,970 scanners in 2001, or 17.4 per million population, compared with 331 in the United Kingdom, or 5.6 per million population.[24]

Just over half of all U.S. machines are located inside hospitals, a relationship that has changed only slightly in recent years.[25] The procedure rate in the United States—63,200 exams per million of U.S. population—was nearly five times the rate in England—12,874 per million.[26]

Cost

MRI equipment is quite costly—approximately $1.5 million for new machines and lesser prices for refurbished, older models, with the exact price varying by age and condition. Because the heart of an MRI machine is a heavy superconducting magnet that generates powerful magnetic fields, additional costs are often necessary to insulate the facility and reinforce floors. Taking all costs into account, total U.S. costs in 2001 were an estimated $3.4 billion.[27] Information on costs of MRI in Britain comes from only a few case studies.[28] Estimated outlays in England totaled $257 million in 2001.[29]

Costs and Trade-offs

In a budget-limited health system, each service must compete with all others for available funds. This rule applies to radiology in the National Health Service. Two decades ago, radiology usually meant common x-rays; CT scanners were new and little used. At that time, the British could have matched U.S. availability and use of these devices at little total cost—an estimated $80 million, or less than 1 percent of hospital expenditures.[30] The decision not to spend the money almost certainly reduced the quality of care.

A Growing Gap

By century's end, the quantity and quality of CT scanning capacity in the United Kingdom had greatly increased. MRI had come on-line, and PET services were available in a few places. But the number of medically indicated applications of diagnostic and interventional radiology had expanded so greatly that the difference between capacity and potential use had widened. The relative gap in service capacity between the United States and the United Kingdom was somewhat reduced from what it had been two decades earlier, but in absolute terms the gap had widened enormously. Two leading London teaching hospitals had to manage with one CT scanner each, while similar hospitals of corresponding prestige in the United States routinely had several.

Even so, British radiologists consulted for this study all reported that the paucity of machines constrains care less than does the lack of trained personnel and sufficient budget to keep available machines running. One radiologist complained, "At the hospital I was at, there were MR and CT machines sitting idle most evenings, even though there were emergencies, but there was not staff to run them."

This problem originated, in part, from an acknowledged mistake. The NHS and medical schools failed to anticipate the sharply increased demand for radiological services and trained too few radiologists. The widespread inability to fill radiological positions at hospitals was the result. The president of the Royal College of Radiology estimates that 10–20 percent of the consultant radiology posts are unfilled.[31] If one allows for vacancies in what in the United States is called "house staff," the overall situation may be even worse. According to another radiologist, "In the area I lived in, in London, the hospital has eight posts for radiologists. Only one was filled. There was only one trained radiologist there for a hospital that should have had eight. . . . And then, it wasn't a poor part of London. It's sort of middle to upper class in terms of wealth. So, those peripheral London hospitals have real difficulties in recruiting staff." Yet another radiologist suggested that the guideline that women between the ages of fifty and sixty-five should be screened every third year for breast cancer intensified the shortage of radiologists and led to limits on the availability of radiology for other uses.

Staff shortages force British facilities to rely on radiographers, rather than physicians, to read films. The NHS standard is that every film should be read by at least two people, one of whom should be a physician. Radiologists admit that failure to meet this standard is common. One radiologist reported that thousands of films at the facility where he had worked were never read at all. Because of meager staffing, British radiologists are unable to specialize in particular organ systems to the degree that is common in the United States. One British radiologist with experience in the United States commented:

> In the States, there's much greater subspecialization, partly because there are many more people in radiology. . . . If you go to Mass General . . . you're going to see different color lines on the floor—green, red, white, blue—and . . . all of these are all of the various subdepartments in radiology. A long time ago, when I was there for the first time, I counted seventy-eight staff, and there are many more

now. At that time, we had something like twelve. So, because there are many more radiologists, you get subspecialization by organ systems. . . . You're going to get chest radiologists, GI [gastrointestinal] radiologists, neuroradiologists, and what have you. In this country, there are recommendations that people should subspecialize largely on an organ system basis, but that happens only every now and then.

Effects on Quality

Repeated interviews produce a composite picture in which British radiologists believe that they are simply unable to provide high quality care for everyone. Rather than addressing the shortages, some practitioners arrange to have patients examined with ultrasound, rather than MRI or CT, a procedure that is adequate for some purposes but less satisfactory for others. Waiting lists are the most visible manifestation of shortages. According to official guidelines, all cancer patients requiring scans are to receive them within two weeks. But patients with conditions that are merely painful often wait much longer. According to one radiologist, "We were running big, long waiting lists. But, in practice, there were only certain types of diseases where you could wait ten months or two years for your MR or your CT scan. Lumbar back problems, knee problems. If it was a case of cancer, some other solution had to be found." Another radiologist made the same point with different emphases:

> The government has decreed that any patient suspected, *seriously* suspected, of having cancer must be sorted out . . . within fourteen days. That is, if someone thinks he has lung cancer, well, he will have been through a CT scanner. He will have had all of his bloods done. He will have had absolutely whatever else, so that the diagnosis can be made within fourteen days. And then the treatment can begin. And sometimes we have problems reaching that target. . . . If he's an outpatient, then we're sometimes a bit pressur[ed] to make sure that he gets whatever he needs within fourteen days. . . . But for seriously ill, or *possibly* seriously ill, patients, all the stops are pulled out. . . . We have this national fourteen-day target. And we all struggle to meet it. [Emphases added.]

While the shortage of diagnostic radiology can generate lengthy waits for scans for patients with non-life-threatening conditions, the shortage of interventional radiologists can produce more serious outcomes. When asked what criteria are used to screen candidates for interventional radiology, one physician answered bluntly,

> Lottery. . . . Near St. Thomas's [a major London teaching hospital] is a district general hospital. You're admitted with a complete . . . inability to swallow [because of a narrowing due to cancer], then you won't get an esophageal stent, a tube in the gullet that will open that narrowing, today or tomorrow or for the next two weeks, because there's no radiologist there that can do the procedure. How do I know that? Well, it happens to be one where they referred me the patient to do. And the reason for the referral is that there is nobody there that can do the procedure. And that patient has not been able to eat anything for two weeks and wouldn't be able to eat anything for another two weeks, because the one radiologist that can do the procedure in that hospital is on vacation. That's just silly. I mean for basic things, it should just not be possible to deprive someone of this basic care.

Who undergoes "lottery rationing" depends in part on where one lives, as facilities are unevenly distributed across the nation. This situation is analogous to but much starker than that in the United States, where the rate of surgery in an area depends in part on how many surgeons practice in that area. In the United States, however, the primary concern is not undersupply in areas with fewer surgeons than average. The major worry is physician-induced demand—an excess of surgery in areas particularly well supplied with surgeons. Access to radiology in Britain may also depend on whom one knows—not in any overtly venal sense but in quite understandable human terms, as illustrated by another comment from the aforementioned radiologist:

> The staff didn't put up with this nonsense. So there was a bypass mechanism. If you had staff who needed a scan, they got it in a sensible time, and the staff's relatives would also bypass the whole system and get a scan done for them. . . . So, if you wanted something done, had no money, it was best to have a relative in the hospital system who generated some goodwill, so that, again, they could bypass the waiting list and so on and get done pretty quickly.

Given the lack of radiology capacity in the NHS, money counts because it enables patients to buy scans privately. This situation raised the possibility that radiologists, like surgeons, might manipulate waiting lists to enhance private patient income. All British radiologists consulted for this study denied that any such manipulation occurs. Why? Not, the respondents replied, because radiologists are more virtuous than surgeons but because backlogs are so sizable that physicians who work privately have all the work they can handle without the need to manipulate anything.

Physicians' Responses

Attitudes of British radiologists differ systematically from those of U.S. physicians regarding the need for and desirability of CT and MRI scans. In U.S. emergency rooms, CT scans have become routine. In the largest hospital in the Washington, D.C., metropolitan area, for example, triage nurses routinely prescribe CT scans before physicians have even seen patients. In all, about one-third of all emergency room patients in that hospital are scanned.[32]

The reactions of British radiologists to such free use of CT scanning vary. One radiologist, who acknowledged that the United States was way ahead of Britain in emergency room radiology, admitted chagrin that only in leading British trauma centers was scanning capacity routinely available at all times. Others expressed the view that U.S. physicians scanned more people than is medically or economically warranted. Once again, it is unclear to what extent these differences reflect fundamental views on how to practice medicine or are a rationalization of resource scarcity, or perhaps some of both.

The shortage of radiological capacity probably influences physicians' referral patterns and diagnostic criteria. When asked whether every patient who "needs" a CT scan gets one, the responses of three radiologists revealed the subtle interplay between medical standards and resource availability. One responded, "I think we do everything that we can do . . . I mean, again, we would tailor it that we would use ultrasound wherever we possibly could, because of cost and time and patient comfort. And we would only use CT where we have to."

A second invoked cost explicitly: "You'll find that in the United States, [CT is used for] many procedures that we would do here under ultrasound guidance simply because it's easier to get one's hands on ultrasound because it's cheaper. . . . Now some of those patients that we would have treated with ultrasound would have been treated more easily and more quickly under CT guidance. There's no question about that."

And according to a third radiologist, who had become quite disillusioned,

I only really had to mention the ten-month waiting list and then that's the end of numerous conversations I had. . . . That was a very good way of blocking them. Also I spent a lot of time trying to fob people off—they wanted an MR—trying to get the same result with an ultrasound or a plain [x-ray]. And, again, that was the end of some conversations. . . . And then after some GPs rang a number of times on this, they didn't bother me again, really, when I was giving them this absurd notion of waiting a year or two. . . . The physician also knew that they had to come up with some other solution to get the radiology or some other way of getting it.

The subtle interplay of medical criteria, cost, and availability also comes through in published research. One article acknowledges that a lack of CT capacity delayed diagnosis but claimed that no patient died "as a direct result" of not having had a CT scan.

There are many reasons why it is necessary to scrutinize requests for CT. One important reason is to avoid inappropriate exposure to ionising radiation. . . . Furthermore, many radiology departments in the U.K. have a fixed budget; thus, they cannot afford the marginal costs of performing more whole-body CT investigations than the allocated budget for CT allows. . . . Whatever methodology is used, no health care system can sustain an exponential use of imaging. . . . Thus radiology departments may be forced to develop some form of rationing for CT requests. . . . There is a perceived, although unproved, notion that clinicians may be more selective in their referrals if they know that their requests are closely scrutinised.[33]

Sensible Savings or Foolish Frugality?

That the scarcity of machines, staffing, and money has reduced availability, eroded quality, and influenced clinical standards of therapy seems inescapable. What is unclear is whether the large difference between British and U.S. spending on radiology reflects a sensible decision on how to allocate scarce medical resources. Although the anecdotal testimony of most British physicians interviewed for this book suggests significant loss of potential benefits, not all agree, and quantitative measures of impact on patient outcome are scarce to nonexistent.

A formal framework for evaluating the worth of improvements in diagnosis helps illuminate the problem. U.S. analysts have suggested that there are at least six ways in which to evaluate improved technology, such as diagnostic imaging.[34] First, does the test perform as intended in a physical sense? For example, can a newer CT scanner distinguish tumor from normal tissue more effectively than an older model did? The second level of evaluation refers to diagnostic accuracy: is the test sensitive and specific? (See note 1.) For example, does a stress test accurately show heart disease when it is present and clearly indicate its absence when it is not? Third, does the test alter the clinician's diagnosis? When simple methods work, sophisticated techniques may add nothing but cost. Fourth, does the test affect the patient's treatment? Accurately diagnosing a condition for which no effective treatment is available has little value. Fifth, do the test and associated changes in treatment improve patient health? Finally, what are the social consequences of the test as measured, for example, by cost effectiveness when compared to another procedure?

Evaluations of the first and second types are most common. A count of studies of magnetic resonance spectroscopy for brain tumors through 2004 revealed that eighty-five level-one studies and eight level-two studies had been performed, but only two level-three studies, two level-four studies, and no level-five or level-six studies. Yet it is level-five and level-six studies that are most relevant for the decisions of the NHS or any other group, private or public, responsible for administering limited health care budgets.

To further complicate matters, the findings of each of the six types of studies of efficacy are highly specific to particular illnesses. CT or MRI may significantly improve diagnosis or treatment of one type of cancer but not another. Simply showing that a new machine produces sharper images in less time than an older machine means little. For example, imaging can identify whether a patient is suffering from the early stages of Alzheimer's disease or some other form of dementia. But the treatment is the same in either case and produces only small benefits and negligible negative side effects. For that reason, the test is not worth the cost, even though it is diagnostically accurate. In still other cases, imaging is acknowledged to produce benefits, but the benefits are small relative to cost. Audiologists frequently prescribe an MRI for patients with hearing loss because there is a small chance—about 1 in 100,000—that the problem stems from an acoustic neuroma, a tumor that is ordinarily treatable and that the test will reveal.[35] U.S. physicians will often prescribe the test. British physicians said they seldom would.[36]

These two examples suggest the difficulties that planners face within a budget-constrained system. One stems from the specific nature of judgments about the value of imaging, which varies widely and is highly specific to particular conditions. Second, the answers require many costly studies, each of a particular condition, to produce the information on whether the test improves patient outcomes at reasonable cost. Few such studies have been carried out relative to the large number of discrete medical conditions. The lack of such studies means that everyone is flying blind—or, at least, with obscured vision. Planners administering a limited budget do not know how many or what kinds of machines to buy or how extensively to staff them. And physicians do not know for which conditions the new equipment will produce demonstrable improvements in patient outcomes. Every British radiologist interviewed for this book expressed the view, usually with caution and invariably with courtesy, that the United States wastes a lot of money on diagnostic equipment and tests that produce little or no benefit to patients. They also indicated that the British spend too little on imaging, with the result that physicians often lack the information to provide patients life-saving or pain-relieving care.

The problem that the British face in deciding how much to spend on diagnostic and interventional radiology crystallizes a larger problem that will confront any health system seeking to limit spending on well-insured patients. Such rationing eventually requires the denial of some beneficial diagnoses and therapies—but which diagnoses and which therapies? To answer this question requires a vast and ever-growing quantity of sophisticated and costly research on which procedures yield which benefits for particular conditions in patients with particular biological characteristics or medical history. Because the research itself is costly, the same rationing principle applies to deciding how much research is worth doing. Not all will pass the test of being cost effective. Currently, however, the potential body of useful information on efficacy is a vast, unexplored continent. In these circumstances, decisions about how much should be spent on radiology—like those concerning most other health technologies—must be made without good research. Those seeking to draw large sums from a limited health budget usually bear the burden of proof to show that the proposed outlay justifies sacrifice of other goods that the money could buy.

For the British to have achieved U.S. service levels for CT, MRI, and PET scanning would have required an increase of approximately £1.7 billion, or nearly 7 percent of the 2001–02 National Health Service hospital budget of £25 billion.[37] A radiologist with experience in both the United States and the United Kingdom put the budgetary problem concretely:

> How much do you put into radiology? One of the points about radiology departments is that they are actually big employers and they're big spenders. . . . You have to pay your technologists, all your booking clerks, goodness knows what else, as opposed to a dermatology department that might only have four or five people. So, there may be 80 or 100 people [in radiology]. Also, they're the only department in the hospital that orders items of equipment costing $1–2 million. . . . So, balancing radiology needs versus needs of, say, dermatology or rheumatology or something can be quite difficult.

Even if radiology is actually the sum of many separate smaller services and is therefore less monolithic than this observation suggests, the fact remains that smaller and less costly services would be justified in claiming that small additions to radiology would be sufficient to fund major increases in other forms of care.

CHAPTER SIX

Rationing and Efficiency

Health care rationing can be done efficiently or inefficiently. This chapter explains the principles that must apply to ensure that whatever is spent on health care yields the largest possible overall benefits. Chapter 8 will raise questions about whether the U.S. political and health care systems are well designed to achieve this outcome.

Some Basic Principles

People are usually assumed to spend their incomes to get as much satisfaction from them as possible. In the jargon of economics, free consumer choice is assumed to be "efficient." Efficiency means that consumers cannot improve their overall satisfaction by buying less of something and more of something else. If producers charge prices that just cover production costs, the value consumers place on each purchase at least equals the cost of producing it.

Health care consumption is not likely to be efficient in this sense. The cause of the inefficiency, paradoxically, is insurance. Insurance, public or private, pays most of the direct costs of health care. Sick people therefore have *economic* incentives to seek any care the benefit from which exceeds the small part of production cost they bear. Such other influences as the advice of physicians or other health professionals also affect the demand for care. But when providers are paid a fee for service rendered, as is common in the United States, they have financial incentives to see that patients receive at least as much care as they want. For these reasons, freely acting health care consumers and providers will tend to seek and receive some care for which the private benefit is less than the value of the goods used to produce it. That is, consumption of health care is unlikely to be efficient.[1]

Every nation with widespread health insurance must find some way to regulate how much it spends on medical care and determine which services to buy. Arrangements may be permissive, as they are in the United States, or highly restrictive, as they are in Great Britain. Whether Britain or the United States spends more or less than it "should" is potentially the subject of endless debate. Health care arguably provides social benefits— a sense of well-being and comfort that accrues to people other than the patients who directly consume it. Social and private benefits combined may exceed production cost, even when private benefits are low. Those who believe such social benefits are considerable may regard quite large amounts of national spending as right and proper. Even identifying the benefits of a commodity whose market price is not an indication of its value to consumers is inevitably somewhat arbitrary.

Spending on medical care varies among nations for many reasons. Rich nations spend more than poor ones do.[2] The United States is richer than the United Kingdom. For that reason alone, U.S. health care spending would be expected to exceed that in the United Kingdom. Still, the United States spends far more than income differentials alone would indicate. The United States compensates physicians far better relative to average earnings than does the United Kingdom.[3] Furthermore, administrative costs in the United States far exceed those of other countries. In addition to differences in income and price, tastes for health care may also vary.

Efficiency

Using resources efficiently is important whether spending is high or low.[*] Does Great Britain use resources efficiently in the sense that it derives as much medical benefit as possible from its relatively modest health care expenditures? Do the differences in the amounts of various forms of care that Britain provides relative to the United States make medical sense? Medical resources are efficiently used when a given total expenditure

---

[*]The material covered in this section is somewhat technical. Readers may skip to the next section on benefit curves without loss of continuity.

cannot be reallocated to alternative kinds of care to achieve an improved medical outcome. To satisfy this condition requires at least five kinds of efficiency.

—*Insurance efficiency* means that insurance should protect people from the risks that cause greatest financial disruption and economic discontent.

—*Medical efficiency* means that the mix of services should produce the greatest possible medical benefit.

—*Distributional efficiency* means that services should be distributed among people to best satisfy a nation's values and preferences.[4]

—*Production efficiency* means that a given quantity of health services should be produced with the fewest possible resources.

—*Dynamic efficiency* means that incentives for technological change should properly encourage scientific advance and the emergence of cost-effective health technology.

This chapter explains how the concept of efficiency bears on medical care and why a nation that curbs medical spending should not curtail all services equally. It then reports estimates of how much of the difference between British and U.S. expenditures stems from the technologies reviewed in the preceding chapters. Chapter 7 evaluates British decisions about which services to curtail, using this standard of efficiency and judgments based on medical effectiveness and social priorities.

Insurance Efficiency

Insurance provides benefits and imposes costs. The principal benefit is protection against the risk of large and burdensome financial losses. The costs take two forms: administrative overhead and encouragement of consumption of services that cost more to produce than they are worth to consumers. Insurance improves welfare only when benefits from the protection against financial risk outweigh the excess of costs over benefits for services that would not be demanded in the absence of insurance and added administrative costs. For these reasons, insurance usually covers items that are individually or cumulatively costly, such as hospital bills or prescription drugs, but it normally does not cover inexpensive items, such as over-the-counter cold medications.

Insurers can use financial devices to hold down demand in various ways, such as narrowing the range of covered services, requiring the insured to pay some initial sum before coverage kicks in, requiring the insured to pay part of costs even after coverage begins, and capping total payments. These steps hold down premiums by increasing patients' exposure to financial risk at time of illness and thereby hold down demand for care. Insurers may also curtail the cost of care administratively by various means. They may deny payment unless prior authorization for care is granted, pay for care only if it is rendered by certain providers, and create red tape, for example, by delaying payment or requiring lengthy waiting times for appointments. Efficient insurance plans produce the highest possible welfare for the insured, given total insurance costs.

Medical Efficiency

Medical efficiency requires that every medical service actually offered produce larger expected benefits per dollar of total cost than any medical service not provided. Imagine a calculation showing the "expected social value" per dollar of expenditure on different forms of health care provided to each patient. A physician undertakes a medical procedure because it has some probability of improving the clinical outcome for a patient. The benefit from the procedure is the social value of the distribution of all possible clinical outcomes, including adverse events, weighted by the value placed on those outcomes by the patient, the patient's family, and sometimes society at large. Benefits may be tangible—for example, the reduced risk for others of contracting a disease when a person is inoculated or given antibiotics—or intangible—for example, the broadly experienced sense of security or justice when the poor receive care for some painful or life-threatening condition.

Distributional Efficiency

Few subjects provoke more passionate and often angry debate than do efforts to decide whether the value of care for different people depends on their personal characteristics or circumstances. Is it equally important to cure the illness of a parent with small children and that of a single person without family obligations? To cure the illness of children, nonaged adults, and the elderly? Of both millionaires and paupers? Of welfare recipients as well as the gainfully employed? Such considerations, as noted in chapter 2, have played a prominent part in the allocation of the National Health Service (NHS) budget among health regions and, more recently, among primary care trusts. The NHS has recently taken on an additional and far more challenging task—that of reducing disparities in health outcomes.

A nation may dodge these questions by paying for all beneficial health care for everyone, but the cost of such avoidance is high, if not already unaffordable. Once a nation explicitly limits total health care spending and thereby denies someone beneficial care, it implicitly places different values on the health outcomes of different people. A health care system that permits disparities in access to health care to be correlated with wealth or income sanctions the resulting inequalities, at least implicitly. Analysis has shown that it is impossible to combine ethical judgments unambiguously into a single collective valuation showing how health care should be distributed. But this fact cannot repeal the inescapable conse-quences of limiting health care spending. Nor does it immunize those judg-ments or the people who make them from moral or political evaluation.

Production Efficiency

Production efficiency requires that a given product be produced with the fewest resources possible. If more resources than necessary are used, over-all efficiency is impossible because other production methods would enable greater total output. In the case of health care services, this condi-tion means, for example, that physicians should not do what nurses can do equally well. It means surgery should be avoided if less costly medical management will produce equal benefits. If one intervention is much more costly than another but even slightly more effective, the decision on which to use is not a judgment about production efficiency but about how much society is prepared to pay to buy the improved outcome.

Dynamic Efficiency

The net benefits from new medical technologies dwarf their costs, on the average.[5] At the same time, there is also abundant evidence that insurance generates static inefficiency, in the sense that some medical services cost more to produce than their benefits are worth at each point in time.[6] What is not known is whether the same payment system that results in excessive provision of care also promotes beneficial scientific advance. This gap in knowledge is critical because short-term waste may promote investments that ultimately generate highly beneficial scientific advances. Financial incentives that influence the current provision of care also shape research and discovery.[7]

Benefit Curves

One can think of efficiency in terms of medical gain per dollar of ex-penditure. Doing so is necessary if one wants to compare the benefits of different medical services—magnetic resonance imaging versus coronary artery surgery, for example. Gain is the medical benefit expected from the procedure as valued by each patient who undergoes the procedure and by others who may be affected by changes in the patient's status. Such comparisons do not imply that one is placing a money value on the benefits of health care. It does mean that, at least subjectively, one is willing to compare the value of diverse services producing very different effects.

Imagine that one has measured such values for all applications of each particular medical service, calculated the value per dollar spent on that service, and ranked benefits per dollar spent from highest to lowest. The graph showing these benefits would depict how fast the expected value per dollar spent declines from the most to the least beneficial application of each service. If one constructed such benefit curves for all services, one would be able to compare benefits across services as well. Of course, clinical outcomes are uncertain, and people generally like to avoid risk. Accordingly, the cost of such uncertainty would be part of the valuation.[8]

Nonmedical factors, such as patients' ages, their underlying health or family responsibilities, and perhaps their social position may influence the valuation of benefits. For some dread diseases, such as cancer, a society may invest heavily, even when the prospects for recovery or improvement are slight, because its members derive comfort from a sense that everything possible is being done or from the delusion that they are still in control.

Figure 6-1 shows hypothetical benefit curves for three procedures. The shapes differ and are arbitrary. Although none has an empirical basis, the contrasting shapes may be taken to represent the benefits of various services. "Units of care" are defined as the quantity of a service that can be purchased for $1.00. The height of the curves indicates benefits per dollar spent. Some procedures—splinting broken bones, for example—produce large benefits for a clearly defined population, but none for anyone else (procedure A). Other procedures—magnetic resonance imaging (MRI), for example—result in large benefits for a few people and small benefits for a very large population (procedure B). Still other procedures may produce gradually decreasing benefits as expenditures on them increase (procedure C). The curves extend various distances along the x-axis, signifying that widely varying amounts are spent on various forms of care. Curve C crosses the x-axis, indicating that procedure C is overused in the sense that some applications actually cause harm. Over time, new benefit curves appear as procedures proliferate, and old curves

Figure 6-1. *Three Hypothetical Benefit Curves under Different Degrees of Health Care Rationing*[a]

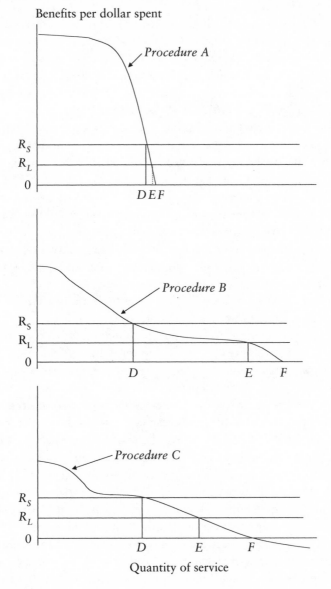

Benefits per dollar spent

Quantity of service

a. R_L, light rationing; R_S, severe rationing; OF, all medically beneficial care is provided; OE, service level at which benefits exceed R_L; OD, service level at which benefits exceed R_S.

may shift position as medical skills improve and new uses for old technologies are found. The growing value of computed tomography and MRI illustrate this phenomenon.

If all medically beneficial, but no harmful, care were provided, the quantity of care would be indicated by line OF as shown for procedures A–C in figure 6-1. Based on the length of OF, the most money would be expended on procedure B; the least, on procedure A. If OF is available for all services and if all uses yield positive expected benefits, rationing does not occur. This level of service is *full provision*. If health care is to be rationed, in the sense that some beneficial care is not provided, one must decide what allocation of outlays will produce maximum medical benefit. Note that this problem exists even if one believes that it is wrong to weigh cost when human health is involved.

It is essential to realize that no commodity for which people have to pay themselves is consumed up to the point of *full provision*. Rational consumers balance the value of spending money on one good rather than another and stop consumption when benefits are positive and roughly equivalent per dollar spent. Almost no one is rich enough to buy goods to the point where additional outlays yield no benefits at all. But, in the case of health care, a fully insured person is in essentially that position, because additional consumption costs nothing.

If health care spending is to be reduced, if all conditions for efficiency are satisfied, and if the benefit curves are regarded as fixed—that is, if technology and tastes are unchanging—then benefit curves such as those drawn in figure 6-1 would indicate which services should be cut back and by how much.[9] For example, suppose that services are to be curtailed, but only slightly, so that no service producing benefits less than R_L (for "light rationing," as shown in figure 6-1) is to be made available. In that event, the quantity spent on each of the hypothetical procedures should decline, but by widely different proportions. The reduction is indicated by the distance from OF, for full provision, to OE, the service level at which benefits exceed R_L.[10] The amount spent on procedure A, for example, should decline negligibly, that spent on procedure B should decline proportionately more, and that on procedure C, most of all. If rationing were more severe so that only services providing benefits greater than R_S (for severe rationing) were to be offered (OD on the x-axis), service A would still be curtailed negligibly (OD versus OF), but procedure B should now be curtailed proportionately more than procedure C.

Whatever the expenditure, however, three central points emerge. First, rationing by reducing each service proportionately is mindless and is normally extremely inefficient. Efficient allocation of limited resources is possible only if all care that yields benefits greater than some minimum is available and no care that promises benefits smaller than that minimum is provided. Such a policy typically implies reducing different procedures by widely varying proportions. It also suggests that the choice of which services to curtail the most may depend on the intensity of rationing.

Second, if resources are limited, not all savings should be sought through reduced quantity. Some quality reductions will likely be required for efficiency. Managers of battlefield hospitals understand that releasing patients sooner than is medically optimal or neglecting some patients altogether may save lives by freeing doctors and nurses to concentrate on those patients who stand to gain most. The fact that hard-pressed municipal hospitals do not provide care up to the standards of university-based teaching hospitals may be evidence of inefficiency, but it may also be a rational way for hospital administrators to respond to differences in resource availability. British hospitals and physicians, likewise, may well be behaving rationally in curtailing the quality as well as the quantity of care. U.S. hospital administrators and physicians could not escape these trade-offs if confronted with severe budget constraints. As Alan Williams put it, "Only when we can be satisfied that the most valuable thing that we are not doing is less valuable than the least valuable thing that we are doing, can we be sure that we are being efficient in the pursuit of welfare."[11] The Williams principle means that some rationing will improve welfare to the extent that resources are shifted from health care that yields few or no benefits to other uses where benefits are positive.

When people have well-ordered preferences among all commodities, are well informed, and behave rationally, benefit curves can be drawn not just for medical care but for all goods and services. The demand for medical services, however, is not a simple expression of the value patients place on them. Patients, who often have little understanding of the benefits that different kinds of care can be expected to yield, depend on health care professionals to act in their interest.[12] No payment system perfectly encourages providers to act faithfully as patients' agents. Fee-for-service compensation encourages providers to render too much care. Conversely, capitation can cause caregivers to stint—and salary provides no incentive for additional effort. Medical ethics exist in part to align providers' and patients' incentives. In a resource-constrained system, providers willy-nilly become society's agents, acting collectively to determine which patients receive how many medical benefits.

Thus providers in a resource-limited system, such as that in Great Britain, face inescapable conflicts among their own interests, those of their patients, and that of society. On the one hand, the dictates of medical ethics and personal professional incentives lead them to serve faithfully as agents for their patients and to advance their own careers. On the other hand, their social responsibility as health care administrators forces them to consider how best to distribute resources among all services and all patients.

Health Expenditures in the United States and Britain

All health systems ration care to some degree, in the sense that not everyone receives all beneficial care. But the severity of budget limits in Britain has produced more pervasive limitations than exist in the United States. First, as noted earlier, the difference in per capita health care expenditures is a key indicator of the severity of British constraints. In 2002 per capita national health care spending in the United Kingdom was 37 percent of that in the United States. This ratio almost certainly misrepresents differences in the availability of care. First, official statistics include items that are not well correlated with patient care, including administration and research. Official statistics understate outlays on these activities in both nations but by amounts that are difficult to estimate precisely. Successful research leads to new knowledge that can be applied not just in the country that supported the research. The U.S. system of administering health care is notoriously cumbersome. Official statistics indicate that on a per capita basis, the United States spends about one-fourth as much on health insurance administration as the United Kingdom spends on all health care—and these statistics exclude administrative costs incurred by physicians, hospitals, and others to bill private and public payers. In addition, U.S. national health care expenditure accounts separately list construction; British accounts do not. While subtracting all of these items understates U.S. spending relative to that of the United Kingdom, this adjustment increases per capita U.K. spending only slightly, to 40 percent of that in the United States.

Second, and more important, both compensation and productivity differ between the U.S. and the U.K. health care systems. Gross domestic product per employed person in the United States exceeded that in the United Kingdom by 25 percent in 2003.[13] The ratio of compensation of U.S. physicians relative to average earners is estimated to be 4.3, compared to 2.5 for U.K. physicians.[14] On the other hand, U.S. health care providers have more capital to work with in both hospitals and outpatient settings, and more capital translates into more services. U.S. physicians, who are mostly paid fees for services rendered, tend to work longer hours than do British physicians, who are mostly paid by salary or flat capitation. In addition, the British purchase drugs centrally and receive discounts on many products. How large these discounts may be is a matter of considerable dispute. Accurately adjusting for the effects on services of relative compensation, productivity differences, and drug discounts has proven impossible. If one arbitrarily assumes that the higher compensation of U.S. physicians and hospital staff more than offsets any productivity advantage, and if one further assumes that the U.S. system produces 25 percent fewer services per dollar spent on physicians, 15 percent fewer services per dollar spent on hospitals, and 20 percent fewer drugs per dollar spent than does the British system, then U.K. residents on average consume just under half the health care services of U.S. residents.

Third, the underlying incidence of illness almost certainly differs from one nation to another. It is impossible to observe these differences directly. All that is visible is the actual incidence of disease or causes of mortality, both of which depend not only on underlying risks but also on the effects of the health care system itself. Take heart disease, for example. While coronary mortality a generation ago was lower in the United Kingdom than in the United States, it is now higher (see table below).[15]

Deaths per 100,000 population

Year	United States		United Kingdom	
	Men	Women	Men	Women
1969	674	261	526	177
1998	203	84	265	97

Source: British Heart Foundation Statistics Database, "Age-Standardised Death Rates."

Even if this shift is attributable to differences in the availability of modern coronary care, it is not clear whether the U.S. population is more or less prone to coronary disease than is the British. Similarly, death from cancer occurs less frequently in the United States than in Britain.[16]

Though not directly observable, the underlying risk of illness bears directly on the severity of constraints on the availability of care that observed differences in spending imply.

One clearly observable risk factor is age. The British population is somewhat older than that of the United States. In 2000, 15.9 percent of the British population was sixty-five or older, compared with 12.4 percent of the U.S. population.[17] Because the elderly typically consume far more health care than do young adults, the age difference suggests that the adjusted expenditure data may slightly understate differences in availability of care.

What Would It Cost to Close the Gap?

Table 6-1 presents estimates of how much it would cost for the British to provide as many of the services examined in preceding chapters as are available in the United States. Where the British provide fewer services than do Americans, U.S. practices are taken to represent "full" care, even in those situations where the U.S. provision is alleged to include low- or no-benefit care. The assumption that all quantity differences represent underprovision in Britain doubtless overstates the amount of quantity rationing there. On the other hand, table 6-1 uses British service costs to measure what it would take to close the gap, and these costs are typically lower—often much lower—than those in the United States. Some part of these cost differences reflects the fact that prices for health resources are lower in Great Britain than in the United States. British wages, for example are lower than U.S. wages, and productivity differences may not correspond to pay differentials. Some part also reflects quality. The British use fewer capital goods and may use fewer or less highly trained staff. The paucity of radiologists and the use of technicians rather than physicians to read test results, as reported in chapter 5, are illustrative. It is impossible to say which bias is larger: the upward bias of assuming all U.S. care is appropriate or the downward bias of assuming that price differences do not denote quality differences.

One very important quality difference between U.S. and British care is wholly ignored in table 6-1. The old quip reported in chapter 4 that in the NHS "you wait to avoid paying or pay to avoid waiting" encapsulates the indisputable fact that waiting is a form of rationing, and it is costly to patients. Table 6-1 makes no allowance for waiting times, which remain longer in Great Britain than they are in the United States. Official

Table 6-1. *Approximate Annual Cost of Increasing Selected Services in Britain to Match United States Levels*

Units as indicated

Service	Added U.K. cost (billions of British pounds)	Added U.K. cost as percent of U.K. spending, 2002[a]	
		Hospital spending	Total health care spending[b]
Stem cell transplantation	0.1	0.4	0.2
Intensive care	4.2	16.5	8.0
Radiology	1.7	6.7	3.2
Coronary artery surgery	1.7	6.7	3.2
Hemodialysis and kidney transplants	0.8	3.1	1.5
Hemophilia factor transfusions	0	0	0
Hip replacement	0	0	0
Outpatient drugs	8.8	. . .	16.8
Total	17.7	33.5	33.0

Sources: Authors' estimates are based on British service costs, which in many cases are well below U.S. costs. Because differences between British service levels and full care are approximations, the estimates are subject to some uncertainty. The drug estimate allows for generally lower drug prices in the United Kingdom. Danzon estimated that drug prices averaged 23.9 percent lower in the United Kingdom than they were in the United States. See Patricia Danzon, "Price Comparisons for Pharmaceuticals: A Review of U.S. and Cross-National Studies, April 1999" (knowledge.wharton.upenn.edu/papers/154.pdf [June 2005]).

a. Department of Health spending on hospital care in 2002 was £25.4 billion; spending on total health care was £52.5 billion.

b. Total health care spending includes hospital care, other medical care, and community health care.

accounts wholly ignore the cost of waiting. By spending more tangible resources to reduce queues, the British would avoid a large cost that they now incur. By analogy, a decision to save money by rationing care in the United States would generate costs invisible to private and public budgets, but not less real for this intangibility, in the form of waiting and inconvenience.

Subject to these qualifications, the British would have to raise *hospital* spending by one-third to provide the specific services examined in this book at U.S. levels. These services represent only a part of the services rendered in any hospital. Chapter 4 examines coronary artery surgery and angioplasty but not valve replacement. It compares rates of replacing hips but not knees. Chapter 5 compares the use of computed tomography and MRI but not positron emission tomography and conventional x-rays. Table 6-1 ignores the impact of the relative paucity of intensive care beds in Britain on the rates of various forms of surgery, which several British physicians said was significant. Differences in expenditures on or use of laboratory tests of various kinds are unexplored. This omission is important because tests are cumulatively costly but individually relatively inexpensive. Stinting on the frequency of blood and other tests is a smoothly variable decision with smoothly decreasing quality as test frequency diminishes.

Table 6-1 also includes a crude estimate of the difference in the use of prescription drugs by outpatients. This comparison is based on U.S. and British data on expenditures adjusted for the estimated average difference in drug costs incurred for outpatients in the United States and Great Britain. Once these drug costs are included in the equation, the British would have to raise *total* health care spending—in and out of hospitals—by just under one-third to match U.S. use of both prescription drugs and the specific services examined in this book.

These comparisons underscore how budget limits have forced curtailment of established services as well as the specific technologies treated here. Budget limits as severe and protracted as those in Britain must inevitably cause significant economies in the provision of a broad range of medical services. But the gaps in provision of some new technologies are disproportionately large. The rapid advances in diagnostic and therapeutic procedures and the concomitant escalation in health care spending have outpaced income growth for at least half a century in both the United States and the United Kingdom.

From 1990 through 2001, health care spending grew at an even faster rate in the United Kingdom than in the United States, but the absolute gap widened because U.S. spending was so much higher to start with. In Great Britain, the reaction of Labour and Conservative governments alike for many years was to "hold the line" and force the NHS to manage with budgets that did not increase as a share of national income. The Blair government reversed that policy. It promised to raise British spending as a share of income to the European average. This decision reflects a judgment that Britain can afford—and its voters want and are willing to pay for—more health care services than previous parsimony would permit. In the United States, spending growth slowed during the 1990s. As a result, concern about "out-of-control" medical spending temporarily abated.

But the resurgence of a rapid increase in health care spending in 2001 rekindled angst about spiraling costs.

Chapters 3, 4, and 5 portray rationing of widely varying intensity. The next chapter examines whether the pattern of rationing found in Great Britain reflects efficient resource use and whether U.S. decisionmakers would be likely to make similar decisions if confronted with similar constraints.

CHAPTER SEVEN

Efficiency and Inefficiency in British Health Care

Efficiency in the use of medical resources requires that all care *not* provided be less valuable than any care that *is* provided.[1] No medical system passes this test. Every country, even those in which services are severely rationed, wastes some resources because of correctable clinical errors that misdirect services to patients who are unlikely to benefit from them. But the evidence reported here confirms that the British system fails the test of efficiency in another sense. While some services are provided up to or near the point at which medical benefits are maximized, whole categories of services receive so few resources that large potential benefits are missed. Reallocation of resources could improve welfare without any increase in total spending. And some increase in health care spending seems likely to more than repay the sacrifice of other forms of consumption, a view expressed in the policy of the Blair government.

Resource misallocation is not new to the British system. In the early 1980s, people with chronic kidney failure died prematurely for lack of dialysis while the lives of patients with metastatic cancer were briefly prolonged at considerable cost. Many hospitals lacked computed tomography (CT) scanners that would have yielded large medical benefits, whereas bone marrow transplantation for several hundred patients a year absorbed enough money to supply many of the missing CT scanners.

Official British policy has recognized the importance of allocating resources efficiently. The National Institute for Clinical Excellence is attempting to compute the cost of extending and improving the quality of life so that resources can be applied to greatest effect. Through a steadily lengthening roster of studies, the institute has sought to determine which procedures yield the biggest benefit per pound spent. The glaring inadequacy of treatment for chronic renal failure has been ameliorated. But new gaps have emerged—in the availability of angioplasty, for example— and old ones persist—for example, in advanced imaging capacity.

Chapter 1 sketched some hypotheses about factors that might influence the allocation of resources to health care in Britain—and, by inference, in the United States should we choose to ration care to the well insured. The observations in chapter 1 and this chapter are, perforce, limited to the few technologies covered here.[2] Readers should judge whether these observations are likely to have general validity.

Acute, life-threatening illnesses are largely exempt from the rationing process in Britain. The payoff from successfully treating a brief but life-threatening illness is large and apparent to all. Furthermore, an acutely ill patient who arrives in an emergency room cannot be denied prompt admission and all available care without imposing insupportable psychological burdens on providers. Once such patients are admitted, the British system, like that of the United States, uses all available resources as long as even a remote chance of returning them to normal or near normal health remains. That said, many services may be simply unavailable, as in the case of angioplasty after heart attacks, and the British acknowledge and U.S. observers have confirmed that the British may treat the elderly or terminally ill more conservatively than would be typical in the U.S. system.

Two decades ago British physicians were asked how they would handle an accident victim whose described injuries were based on those of an actual case admitted to a large U.S. teaching hospital. Respondents were asked to accept that the patient had one chance in a hundred of surviving and that the minimum cost of care would be at least $270,000. These conditions imply that one would expect to spend at least $27 million to save one life. Despite the limitations they face, the British physicians unanimously stated that they would have used all available resources just as their American counterparts had done.[3]

Factors That Seem to Influence Allocation among Technologies

Whether particular treatments will be well or poorly funded depends on medical considerations and social influences that sometimes offset and sometimes reinforce one another. Disentangling the many forces that seem consistent with actual funding decisions made in Great Britain defies rigorous or formal analysis.

Chronic Dialysis

Many patients in the early 1980s died prematurely because the supply of chronic dialysis was inadequate. National Health Service (NHS) budgets hardly grew, rising barely 1 percent a year in real terms. Boosting treatment of chronic kidney failure to U.S. levels would have required freezing real spending by the rest of the NHS for two years, even as the population aged and technology advanced. Lack of access—dialysis centers were located disproportionately in the London region—abetted rationing. So did centralized control over capital expenditure on equipment and trained personnel, which confronted nephrologists with an external constraint to which they had to adjust. The typical general practitioners saw a renal failure case no more often than once every two or three years. As reported in chapter 3, general practitioners came to appreciate the futility of referring patients who were unlikely to be treated and who would die quietly, without extended pain. Furthermore, physicians could rationalize the refusal to treat renal failure patients, who often suffer from comorbidities, such as diabetes. None of these considerations, other than the frequency of comorbidities, is immutable.

In the last two decades, dialysis centers have proliferated. British patients increasingly have ready access to renal replacement therapy. Technical advance has improved the dialysis experience. General practitioners report now that they are unwilling to cut off patients from access to a lifesaving procedure. And the dialysis "community"—patients and providers—has mobilized to lobby for increased resources.

British service levels were once a small fraction of those of most Western European nations. That gap has been largely closed. To be sure, U.S. rates of care continue to exceed those in Great Britain by about the same ratio as they did two decades ago. Differences in epidemiology—most notably from diabetic nephropathy—explain much of the gap, but that a gap remains, particularly in treatment of the elderly, is clear.

The evolution of dialysis rationing is suggestive. A lifesaving technology comes onstream, available at first in only a few centers to which many would-be patients lack ready access. Providers and patients mobilize to increase spending. They succeed in part, but access remains below that of an unconstrained system. In brief, experience with dialysis suggests that recently developed therapies are likely to be more severely rationed than are those that have entered into standard use.

Hemophilia

While gaps in the treatment of chronic renal failure were large and have narrowed, gaps in the treatment of hemophilia were small and have vanished. In contrast to renal failure, the symptoms of hemophilia are blatant and alarming. Two decades ago a major breakthrough in hemophilia treatment had just occurred, but it was then followed by the catastrophe of HIV-contaminated infusions. From this tragedy came further improvements in treatment, as a result of which hemophiliacs now enjoy near-normal life expectancies. Capital investment required for treating hemophilia is minimal.

In the early 1980s, providing every renal failure patient with dialysis when medically indicated would have cost roughly ten times as much as it did to treat all hemophiliacs. By spending a little, the British could forestall the visible devastation and the costly disabilities from hemophilia for which society would have had to pay if care had been suboptimal. Since then the cost of treating hemophilia has risen strikingly—from about $6,000 within the NHS and $5,600 in the United States in the early 1980s, to between $40,000 to $70,000 in the United Kingdom and $50,000 to $100,000 in the United States.[4] Treatment has become more intensive, and blood products have become more costly. The patient population has grown enormously as longevity has increased. Despite these rising costs, hemophilia continues to be treated fully, a policy that contrasts with persistent limits on dialysis. The most obvious explanation is that abandoning an established policy of full treatment is harder than allowing less-than-complete treatment to persist. The willingness to pay what it costs to treat hemophilia may also reflect the emotive force of the stark symptoms of hemophilia compared to the quiet decline associated with renal failure.

Hip Replacement

For decades the thousands of British residents who waited years for hip surgery sullied the image of the National Health Service. Lengthy waiting lists and waiting times persisted although NHS hip replacement rates were close to those in the United States. Chapter 3 explained why more was not spent to shorten those lists and waiting times. But why so much was spent on hip replacements to reduce pain and improve mobility of the elderly while so little was spent on dialysis to save lives has been something of a mystery. One possible reason was unit cost. Dialysis, which had to continue as long as the patient lived, cost twice as much each year as the one-time cost of a new hip that could last many years. Second, patients enjoy a basically normal life after successful hip surgery whereas patients on dialysis suffer complications, inconvenience, and various discomforts. In fact, many patients passively commit suicide by voluntarily stopping dialysis. Finally, failure to replace diseased hips raises costs because untreated hip patients typically require costly nursing care, either at home or in a public institution. Failure to treat renal failure lowers costs because patients with untreated renal failure die, usually quickly, inexpensively, and unobtrusively.

As spending has risen, the Blair government has struggled to expunge the image of long waiting times as the symbol of the NHS. The average time patients spend on waiting lists for hip replacements has been sharply reduced, and the government is committed to ambitious goals for further improvement.

Coronary Artery Surgery

The limitations on treatment of coronary artery disease have persisted almost without change for more than two decades. In the early 1980s, the British performed coronary artery surgery at about one-ninth of the U.S. rate. In 2002 the combined rate of angioplasty and coronary artery surgery in the United Kingdom had risen to roughly 23 percent that of the United States, and yet the absolute gap in treatment had grown enormously. Why?

Even if the American rate is higher than optimal, as seems likely, the British might do many more of these procedures with considerable medical benefit, as British experts acknowledge. Age hardly seems to be a factor. Hip surgery is provided far more generously than are coronary artery surgery and angioplasty to roughly the same age group. Cost is surely a major impediment to full treatment. Provision of coronary artery surgery and angioplasty at U.S. rates would require an increase in the NHS hospital budget of nearly 7 percent. Two other factors may also contribute to the nearly full treatment of hip disease and the severe stinting in coronary care. First, the symptoms of an elderly woman with hip disease, bedridden or barely able to walk, are obvious to others. Those of a middle-aged man with coronary artery disease who must walk slowly to avoid chest pain are not. Furthermore, medications permit most angina patients to look after their personal needs and remain mobile enough not to require nursing or other supportive care. Severe hip disease creates far greater demands. Second, it has been hard to detect the impact of coronary artery bypass surgery and angioplasty on mortality in patients with most types of coronary disease. However, recently published findings on the benefits of angioplasty in terms of averting lasting damage to the heart after coronaries have dramatized the advantages of this costly procedure.[5] British hesitancy to develop the capacity to provide angioplasty and to use drug-coated stents illustrates that resource limits most profoundly affect new procedures whose efficacy is considered unproven.

Stem Cell Transplantation

Stem cell transplantation contrasts with other procedures examined here in that the relative frequency of treatment in Britain has declined sharply, from near parity with that in the United States in the early 1980s to 77 percent of the U.S. rate today. Three conditions may have contributed to the earlier relative parity for this procedure: the youth of bone marrow transplant recipients, the often lifesaving nature of the treatment, and the low aggregate cost, because few patients were suitable candidates for treatment.

In more recent times, changes in two of these conditions have likely contributed to the failure of stem cell therapy in Britain to keep pace with that in the United States. Advances in therapeutic techniques have not only sharply increased the cost of treatment but have also boosted the average age of patients who can be successfully treated. Thus, compared to two decades ago, outlays in the United States are now sixty times higher and in the United Kingdom, more than twenty times higher. Whereas in the early 1980s patients were young and total treatment costs were low, now the typical patient is much older and total treatment costs have become burdensome. U.S. observers would tend to regard the emerging gap in outlays as costs rise as a reflection of British resource constraints. British observers might claim the difference arises from incentives to overtreat under a fee-for-service payment system.

Diagnostic Radiology

Two decades ago, the British lagged behind the United States in radiology. They could have achieved parity at modest cost but chose not to do so. Slowly growing NHS budgets left little financial room for doing more than serve a growing population. The breathtaking technological advances in radiology of the past quarter century were just beginning. Patients had no way to know whether further investigations were medically warranted or not. These circumstances led to the sluggish introduction of new medical technology.

In the first years of the twenty-first century, all of these conditions except the last have changed. Diagnostic radiology has become central to adequate therapy, particularly in determining cancer stages and in planning radiation treatments. A whole new field of interventional radiology has emerged.[6] And the Blair government has initiated large increases in NHS spending. Under these circumstances, the gap in radiology between the United Kingdom and the United States—relatively as large in 2000 as in the early 1980s and absolutely far larger—inspired large investments in new equipment, resulting in a 50 percent increase in CT scanners between 2001 and 2004. Yet the lack of personnel to run the new machines and interpret the resulting images has become a more serious bottleneck than lack of capital, raising concerns about the quality of care. Furthermore, no similar commitment has been made to the newer technology of positron emission scanning. As the NHS has increased purchases of scanners, charitable gifts are reported to have shifted from the creation of new facilities to upgrades and extras.

These developments indicate why introduction of new, capital-dependent medical technologies is particularly sensitive to budget constraints. In the early 1980s, NHS budget growth paid for little more than maintaining services for a growing and aging population. In that environment, funds for the purchase of costly new equipment could be found only by actually reducing traditional services. When constraints are relaxed, hardware manufacturers are able to fill orders quickly even when, as in Great Britain today, personnel bottlenecks, such as the dearth of radiologists, threaten quality.

Intensive Care Beds

One of the defining characteristics of health care rationing in Great Britain is the relative paucity of intensive care facilities. The direct cost of U.S. intensive care units (ICUs) is huge, perhaps 25 percent of the U.S. hospital budget. In addition, the availability of ICU beds is essential for certain types of surgery. British physicians candidly acknowledge that surgeries sometimes cannot be scheduled because an ICU bed is unavailable. Thus the stock of ICU beds indirectly shapes the amount and kind of surgery and general medical practice. Despite the large increase in NHS budgets after 2000, there is little evidence of a major increase in the number of ICU beds.

Terminal Illness

British physicians commented repeatedly that they would discontinue aggressive therapy for the terminally ill earlier than their American counterparts do. They also, and just as repeatedly, asserted that they would elect to stop treatment earlier than Americans do even if their resources were not constrained. This claim undoubtedly reflects cultural traditions and ethical views.

On the other hand, the limitation on intensive care beds, the low rates of coronary revascularization, and other constraints force British physicians to practice triage. The sheer availability of ICU beds in the United States spares American physicians the need to face such hard decisions, even if they might explicitly agree with the values expressed by their British colleagues.

Factors That Seem to Influence Resource Allocation

Certain general principles seem implicit in decisions regarding the technologies described here. Some reflect the influence of administrative arrangements on the allocation process. Others express society's value judgments. Still others seem to be attempts to make the most efficient use of available resources.

Age

If all other factors were held constant, rationing of health care for the elderly would likely be more severe than that for the young. Aggregate data support this prediction. Health expenditures per child in the early 1980s were 119 percent of expenditures per prime-age adult in Britain, whereas in the United States, they were only 37 percent as much.[7] Evolutionary forces have led adults to be protective of children. Cold arithmetic shows that on the average, spending health care resources on the young extends or improves lives for more years than if the same resources are spent on the old.[8] The responsibilities of prime-age adults as parents and earners may override these considerations, but prime-age adults typically make few demands on the health care system. Such offsetting factors seldom apply to the elderly.

Visibility of Illness

Visible misery disturbs observers as well as the sufferer. The patient's family, friends, and casual contacts are made uncomfortable if they must watch severe and untreated suffering. The bleeding joints, swelling, and disabilities of hemophilia stir the emotions of bystanders in a way that the silent pain of angina does not. The tragic situation of hemophiliacs who were infected with HIV by the very blood products used to treat them doubtless reinforced such feelings. Thus it is hardly surprising that in Britain more support is allocated to providing clotting factors for hemophiliacs than to providing bypass surgery or angioplasty for angina patients.

Advocacy

Organized advocates can try to use political pressure, publicity, or charity to obtain facilities and personnel for a particular service. Two decades ago, there was little evidence that advocacy played an important role in shaping allocation decisions in Britain. Other than bone marrow transplantation, no service was significantly increased by the efforts of pressure groups.

The situation in Britain has changed. Nephrologists credit patient groups for helping push up dialysis budgets. In a more diffuse fashion, long waiting lists, a perennial public relations nightmare for the NHS, became a major motivation for increasing total NHS budgets. The growing role of activism by groups of patients is probably linked to a more general trend reported by numerous British physicians: a growing inquisitiveness and willingness of patients to challenge and second-guess physicians, even to sue them. Some greet this trend as salutary and long overdue. Others see it as evidence of unattractive selfish individualism— what they regard as the Americanization of British society.

Aggregate Cost

A service that is expensive per patient may still cost little in the aggregate. In the early 1980s, treatment of hemophilia in Britain seemed to fall into such a category. Fewer than 100 new cases of hemophilia were diagnosed annually. The small aggregate cost of sparing each new cohort the devastation of this illness seemed well worth incurring. The population of hemophiliacs has risen to more than 6,000 as successive cohorts have been spared early deaths. Per patient treatment costs have also increased. Still, the aggregate cost of treatment is just over 0.3 percent of total health care spending. It is doubtful that the policy of full treatment of hemophilia would have become entrenched if new patients numbered several thousand rather than fewer than 100 each year.

Capital and Personnel Controls

New technologies that require dedicated capital equipment or specially trained personnel are easier to control than are technologies that physicians and nurses can apply without special training or supplies. A comparison of the use of CT scanners and total parenteral nutrition (TPN) provides striking confirmation of this premise. In the early 1980s, the newly developed CT scanner was used for a narrow range of imaging tasks. Though slow and of limited applicability, it improved patient care where relevant. Because special equipment was required, CT scanning could be controlled simply by not buying machines. Private charity permitted a few communities to evade official limits. Meanwhile, the British spent as much on total parenteral nutrition (TPN), a novel and quite costly way to provide nutrition to patients incapable of eating, as they did on CT scanners, even though the benefits of TPN were not well documented. TPN required only supplies readily available in hospital pharmacies and could be administered by nurses and physicians without special training. Computed tomography, in contrast, depended on single-purpose capital equipment and trained radiologists and technicians.

In the United States the CT scanner rapidly became ubiquitous. Access was easy and quick in most hospitals and in hundreds and then thousands of independent radiology facilities. Abetted by this availability, physicians found multiple uses for CT scanners, even spawning the new subspecialty of interventional radiology. U.S. physicians now have access to CT and the newer magnetic resonance imaging (MRI) scanners as readily as did British physicians to total parenteral nutrition. The effect is similar: controlling use is now extremely difficult, even in applications where benefits are slight or undocumented.

For many years, British hospitals could not hire consultants without authorization from regional or district health authorities. By refusing to fill positions, the NHS could control the supply of particular services. For example, a hospital without a heart surgeon could not offer coronary bypass surgery. A facility with few radiologists and radiographers cannot remain open on weekends or nights. With increasing autonomy for individual hospitals, this instrument of control has been significantly weakened.

Costs of Alternative Modes of Care

Service levels are likely to be higher if the costs of not treating the patient exceed the costs of active intervention. For example, the costs of coronary bypass surgery and hip replacement are similar. Patients likely to undergo such procedures are of similar age. But the proportion of British patients requiring hip replacements who receive them is far higher than the proportion of heart patients who receive coronary surgery or angioplasty. Untreated hip disease generates larger costs, on the average, than does untreated angina.

Quality versus Quantity

The distinction between quantity and quality in medical care is often fuzzy. A shortage of resources to perform the medically optimal procedure may force physicians to use less effective methods. British cardiologists with limited resources often must rely on thrombolytic (clot-busting) drugs to treat patients who have had heart attacks. These drugs are beneficial but are less effective than angioplasty. Radiologists who lack access to modern scanners may rely on ultrasonography, which is less precise and may be less convenient than CT or MRI scans. It might seem sensible, at least sometimes, to dilute the quality of care in order to extend the quantity. Usually, such corner-cutting is false economy. British decisions seem generally to reflect this judgment. The British, in the opinion of experts, maintain virtually the same standards of quality as do Americans for coronary revascularization, hip replacement, and most other treatments. Cutting corners on surgical interventions would exact a heavy toll of bad outcomes and therefore make little sense.

Understaffing of CT and MRI scanners is an exception to the generalization that the British do not stint on quality. Scans are often read by one trained radiologist and one experienced radiographer, not by two radiologists as is considered optimal by British standards. This particular example of skimping seems to have arisen not from an explicit effort to save money, but from a mistake in training too few radiologists.

Dealing with Resource Limits

British doctors and patients alike have adjusted to severe resource limits that well-insured Americans do not experience. Although spending has increased sharply in recent years, the consequences of financial constraints remain pervasive. British responses to resource limits reflect local conditions and history, but most of their responses would evoke similar behaviors under any budget-constrained system.

The Physician's Way

Binding limits mean that physicians can increase control over resources for their patients only by taking them away from others. The extent to which this game can be played is limited, however. For this reason, British physicians often seem to rationalize, or at least to redefine, medical standards so that they can deal more comfortably with resource constraints.

RATIONALIZATION. Resource limits put doctors in a position that many find awkward. Trained to treat illness, they must stint on care that promises their patients medical benefits. Although such limits may well reflect valid social or political judgments that forgone benefits would cost more than they are worth, few physicians are trained to balance social costs and private benefits. Few enjoy making such trade-offs. Wherever possible, therefore, British doctors seem to seek medical justification for decisions forced on them by resource limits. Faced with tight budget constraints, doctors gradually redefine standards of care so that they can escape the constant recognition that financial limits compel them to do less than their best.

A comparison of physician responses in the early 1980s, when there was virtually no growth in per capita health care spending (after adjustments for aging), with responses in 2004, after a period of rapid spending growth, reveals a paradox. In the 1980s, physicians and other health care providers tried in various ways to make the denial of care seem routine or optimal. Confronted by a person older than the prevailing unofficial age cutoff for dialysis, British general practitioners (GPs) told victims of chronic renal failure or their families that nothing could be done except to make the patients as comfortable as possible in the time remaining. British nephrologists told families of patients who were difficult to handle that dialysis would be painful and burdensome and that the patients would be more comfortable without it. Or they might tell resident aliens from poor countries that they should return home, to be among family and friends who speak the same language and where, yes, the patients would die because dialysis was unavailable. Cardiologists focused on the relatively narrow class of cases in which coronary artery surgery demonstrably increased survival rates or in which anginal pain was disabling. They downplayed this option in cases where pain was less severe.

In each instance physicians asserted that treatment was medically optimal or close to it. They asserted that patients denied care or provided less costly alternatives lost essentially nothing of medical significance. At some level providers must have known that such rationalizations—for the renal failure patient who dies for want of dialysis, for the victim of angina denied pain-reducing care, or for the accident victim whose head injuries were incorrectly diagnosed because a CT scanner was unavailable—were bogus. Even if the services that are curtailed reflect a rational set of *social* judgments about which services should be denied, individual physicians find it hard to cope with the knowledge that an inability to offer care causes *their* patients to suffer. Not all British doctors believed they were providing all potentially beneficial care to their patients. Many realized, as one consultant stated, that they were acting as society's agents in rationing care. Another consultant spoke about the process:

> The sense that I have is that there are many situations where resources are sufficiently short so that there must be decisions made as to who is treated. Given that circumstance, the physician, in order to live with himself and to sleep well at night, has to look at the arguments for *not* treating a patient. And there are always some—social, medical, whatever. In many instances he heightens, sharpens, or brings into focus the negative component in order to make himself and the patient comfortable about not going forward. He states the reason for not going forward in medical terms . . . but that formulation in many instances is in no small part conditioned by the fact that there really aren't enough resources to treat everybody, and there is a kind of rationalization which is, perhaps, influenced by resource constraints.[9]

British doctors seemed simultaneously to want to do more but also to believe that their country could not then afford it. Two decades after the ICU manager at a leading teaching hospital said that "everybody would get bored stiff and the place would be half empty" if there were many more intensive care beds, another physician who practiced at the same hospital expressed similar views.[10] Such thought processes are likely to emerge in any severely constrained health care system as doctors acknowledge limits and seek medical rationales for fiscal necessity so that they can at least halfway believe they are giving their patients medically optimal care.

The need to rationalize seems to have weakened as resource availability has increased. By 2004 the NHS had enjoyed several years of rapid expenditure growth. The government had promised that spending would continue to grow much faster than population and income. Official projections indicated that U.K. spending on health as a share of gross domestic product would approach or surpass the average of the Organization for Economic Development and Cooperation. In that environment, physicians readily acknowledged that spending for many services is too low. They stated that some patients are denied care they should receive because resources are limited. While claiming that conditions had improved, they volunteered that the optimal level of care is higher than currently offered in Britain. They also expressed the view that U.S. provision is probably excessive and that the proper target for Great Britain should be somewhere between current British provision and that in the United States. The freeing up of resources released discontents about inadequacies that in more deprived times had been suppressed.

EXPLOITING CLINICAL FREEDOM. The British profess that doctors, in consultation with their patients, should freely determine diagnoses and treatments. They believe that these decisions should not be second-guessed, except in instances of egregious abuse—and then only by medical colleagues or the courts. This principle can be justified by the importance of factors specific to each case in prescribing treatment and the need for doctors to make dozens of choices a day quickly and decisively.

Under the rubric of clinical freedom, physicians can sometimes divert resources to patients in whom they are interested. However, if physicians are excessively aggressive, thereby diminishing resources available to other patients, then their colleagues may intervene. The British system is almost ideally constructed to control such exploitation of clinical freedom. Power over each hospital's budget rests largely in the hands of the hospital's small cadre of senior physicians, who enjoy lifetime tenure. The consultants' personal finances seldom intrude on debates about allocation of the hospital's budget. Negotiations are said to be marked by compromise and trade-offs born of the recognition that members of this club typically spend all or most of their professional lives in the company of the same colleagues.

For many years, the clinical freedom that GPs working outside the hospital enjoyed posed no threat to the budget. General practitioners had little access to costly tests, and outpatient drugs accounted for little of the health budget. The sharp increase in the clinical importance and financial cost of drugs has raised the stakes of GP autonomy. GPs have the power to violate guidelines for drug usage, but if they do so, they may receive queries from colleagues or NHS officials. And among general practitioner groups, physicians who make use of patented drugs when generics are available may be subjected to critical scrutiny. But the system relies on moral suasion rather than explicit rules or punishments.

SHORT-CIRCUITING DELAYS. Limited resources have long translated into queues. Recent vigorous efforts have reduced average waiting times, but physicians concerned about the timeliness of treatment have long had ways to shorten waits for particular patients. General practitioners who feel that a patient should be seen promptly could telephone the consultant rather than writing a letter. The tone of communications likewise can be used to convey urgency.

THE PROBLEM OF SAYING "NO"—THEN AND NOW. Two decades ago British physicians had to refuse patients treatment more often than is now the case. The middle-aged or elderly patient with renal failure was the prime example. Saying "no" to such patients was never easy, of course, but local internists who persuaded themselves that all patients over age fifty or fifty-five are "a bit crumbly" and therefore unsuitable for care could say "no" with little discomfort. For many older patients with renal failure, local physicians did not even raise the possibility of dialysis. Other physicians thereby protected nephrologists from having to say "no." With the increase in resources for dialysis, local physicians now report that they routinely refer all patients with renal failure. Nephrologists report that they find some way to fit in all patients referred to them. Nonetheless, dialysis rates remain lower than on the continent and much lower than in the United States. Disease incidence may account for some of the difference, but the survival of different standards of care from a time when resources were scarcer seems apparent.

Inertia

Data on rates of revascularization and reports of procedures for screening patients for conditions that predispose patients to heart disease both suggest that severe rationing results in suboptimal care. Research has identified tests that can determine which patients are at risk of developing coronary disease. Drugs are available to slow the progress of disease, and interventions exist to counter identified arterial blockages. But this entire chain of treatment depends on routine screening of people who have reached certain ages and criteria for what test results trigger intervention. At each stage—screening, criteria for treatment, and intervention—British standards have lagged behind those of the United States. It seems likely that, as in the case of dialysis, the system will eventually respond to new technologies, and treatment rates will increase, but resource limits retard this process. Delay has an important virtue: it reduces resource waste on methods that do not pan out. However, tardiness in introducing effective methods also may result in avoidable pain or premature death for patients.

Safety Valves for the Patient

Because patients' treatment preferences differ, government or other authorities may determine how much is to be spent on health care and even how much is spent on broad classes of care, but doctors and patients will have to decide how particular cases will be treated. The diversity of preferences also means that officials must decide how to respond when private citizens who chafe at resource limits seek care outside the system.

The two principal channels for health care outside the controlled system are gifts to charity and purchase of medical care outside the National Health Service. British taxpayers, like their U.S. counterparts, may deduct gifts to hospitals or other public health facilities when determining taxable income. However, in contrast to U.S. practice, the British may not deduct private health expenditures or health insurance premiums. These two options allow British citizens to indulge their preferences by going outside the NHS rather than by demanding more or different health care within it. The availability of private insurance also means that excessively stringent limits on NHS expenditures could threaten the survival of the health service by driving too many people to "go private."

This framework offers what may be the most plausible (if tautological) explanation for the sharp increase in NHS budgets under the Blair administration. The government recognized that an increasingly prosperous citizenry, with expanding awareness of health standards in other nations and willingness to question the high priests of medicine, simply would not stand for limits that their parents had readily accepted. The deductibility of gifts to private charitable organizations and the regulatory policies that permit NHS doctors to practice privately have an important indirect bearing on popular attitudes toward the budget limits imposed on the National Health Service. The more attractive the choices are outside the NHS, the less stake patients have in the NHS or in relaxing the budget limits constraining it.

CHARITY. Charity plays a minor part in British medicine as a whole, but it has been significant in selected fields. A few large hospitals retain endowments from pre-NHS days. Some medical equipment, notably scanners, has been purchased out of donated funds. Private funds have endowed senior consultancies in certain fields, notably oncology, to increase the prestige and visibility of such specialties.

Some lessons emerge from these gifts. First, British donors, like their American counterparts, exhibit the "edifice complex," a preference for giving buildings or equipment over paying for its continued operation and maintenance. For this reason gifts have sometimes enticed or pressured authorities into changing their priorities. The gift of a CT scanner, unaccompanied by funds for staff, supplies, and maintenance, thus burdens the budget of the NHS unit where the scanner is located. Endowing chairs for professors may entail the complementary hiring of junior doctors and other support staff and reserving an appropriate number of beds to which the newly honored appointee will have admitting privileges. Because of such expenses, beneficiaries sometimes decline such gifts if they are unaccompanied by funds for operating or ancillary expenses.

Second, health authorities that anticipate gifts can divert their own resources to other purposes. Anticipated gifts thus may not change priorities but simply add to health spending. The NHS might have invested more and earlier in CT and MRI scanners had private donations not partially filled the gap and were further donations not anticipated.

THE PRIVATE SECTOR. When the public sector does not provide all the health care people want, patients must decide whether to seek it elsewhere. Their willingness to do so depends on how highly they value the services in short supply and how much extra they must personally pay for them. Informed and aggressive patients with adequate wealth or insurance are well situated to access the care or amenities they want outside the controlled system. For example, patients who are willing to pay to see consultants as private patients are likely to be seen more quickly than are those who wait to see consultants through the National Health Service.

Although private care survived under the NHS, there was little of it until the late 1970s when it came to provide a significant part of some forms of health care. Patients could circumvent long waits for elective surgery in aging NHS hospitals by going to newly built private hospitals where they could receive prompt treatment and enjoy such amenities as private rooms. The NHS continued to provide backup protection against serious complications. Patients who needed specialized care unavailable in a private hospital could be moved to an NHS facility. The private sector could not then provide the high-priced and sophisticated care supplied almost exclusively by the NHS.

Private hospitals, sometimes funded by foreign investors and staffed by foreign physicians, now feature increasingly modern equipment. Yet the NHS still usually remains the best place for complex procedures because backup care depends on laboratories and on junior physicians for twenty-four-hour care, all of which involve high-overhead expenses, although some private facilities are reported to meet these standards. Such costly care can be sustained in private facilities only if the demand is high.

Insurance coverage for such care is unlikely to develop in any large way. People at low risk of needing elaborate and costly care are unlikely to pay premiums for private insurance to cover the costs of procedures, such as dialysis, that might be in short supply within the NHS. But if only those at high risk of needing complex services sign up, insurance would be extremely costly. Thus, as a case in point, virtually no dialysis in Britain is performed outside the National Health Service. In 2000 private health care spending (including nonprescription drugs) accounted for only 19 percent of total health outlays in the United Kingdom.[11]

WORKING THE SYSTEM. British physicians describe a sharp change in patient attitudes toward health care and the medical profession. Two decades ago, patients typically took the word of their physicians on a course of action—or inaction. Patients now are reported to question providers and to demand high-quality service more insistently than in the past. Even worse—or better, depending on the respondent—British patients have become increasingly litigious.

Aggressive patients have always had several strategies open to them if they wished to press forward within the system. They could ask physicians to arrange for second opinions, which in most instances, were provided without protest. Patients could try to gain access to specialized services they had previously been denied by going to a hospital emergency room, even that of a major university hospital. The emergency room also provided access to primary care services outside office hours. On rare occasions, patients could penetrate the referral barrier by going directly to the clinic of a specialist. In the time when dialysis was virtually unavailable to the elderly, one leading nephrologist reported that if a patient sat down in the waiting room he or she would probably be seen and a slot found in the dialysis program. A cancer expert confessed that the key to turning down the patient "is not to get eyeball-to-eyeball with him because if you do, there is no way you can actually say no."[12]

EXPLOITING GEOGRAPHY. Medical services are more readily available in London and a few other areas than elsewhere. In the past, waiting times for hip replacement varied widely across regions.[13] Nephrologists emphasize that the availability of dialysis has increased not just because the number of centers has grown but because they are more evenly spread across the nation than in the past. Patients have always been free to travel to areas with short queues or abundant services, but few have done so. Patients are reluctant to leave familiar surroundings and the emotional support of friends and relatives. Extensive research in both the United States and Great Britain finds that proximity to care is a prominent determinant of use.[14]

Why Malpractice Litigation Does Not Mobilize Resources

In a budget-constrained system, the direct effect of successful malpractice litigation is not to increase resources but to redirect them to the successful litigant from other potential beneficiaries. It is possible that successful malpractice litigation beyond some threshold might indirectly pressure the government to expand medical services; however, it is hard to detect evidence that such a threshold has been crossed in Britain. Although the British malpractice docket has expanded greatly in the past quarter century, it remains relatively light by U.S. standards. The number of claims reached 100 for all England and Wales only in 1977 and passed 1,000 only in 1990. The number of suits filed per year exceeded 5,000 from 1995 through 1999 but then fell sharply. By comparison, 86,480 claims were filed in the United States in 2000, approximately three times the British rate after adjustment for population.[15] Despite rates of litigation for which U.S. physicians might pine, British physicians during the late 1980s voiced concern about a malpractice crisis and warned that physicians were being driven to defensive medicine. These concerns were expressed even though the NHS paid all or part of malpractice premiums

for many physicians. The NHS paid the entire premium for general practitioners. It paid for two-thirds of premiums for consultants in the late
1980s and paid for the entire premium starting in 1990. In 1995 the NHS
established its own litigation authority to indemnify NHS groups and
employees for malpractice costs.[16]

The flow and ebb of malpractice litigation in the late 1980s arose in
part from identifiable government regulations and in part from changing
popular and professional attitudes. Proper medical behavior, based on a
court decision handed down in 1957, was "that of a reasonably competent medical practitioner exercising and professing to have that skill."[17]
The meaning of this rule is not entirely clear, as competent medical practitioners routinely err. One practicing radiologist suggested that

> doctors themselves are to blame [for the increase in litigation]
> because those people that acted as advisors to lawyers just simply
> did not point this out [the error inherent in human activity]. . . .
> They would go to court and they put up a chest x-ray . . . and say,
> "There's a cancer. I would expect any competent radiologist to be
> able to see that." And that's true—as a stand-alone statement it
> would be true. But it's also true to say that every single one of those
> experts would have missed just that kind of cancer in the last several
> years, simply because everybody has a miss rate. That was never
> pointed out to the court. And the court just said, "OK, you missed
> it, you pay."

From the early days of the NHS, legal aid was provided to help low-
income citizens bring malpractice cases. In 1996 a report prepared under
the direction of Lord Woolf, then Britain's most senior judge, found that
92 percent of medical negligence claims were funded by Legal Aid from
the government. Less than half the population, only those on income support, qualified for full or partial legal funding. With no evidence that the
poor were disproportionately the victims of medical negligence, the
Woolf report observed that many victims failed to bring claims for errors
because of the cost.[18]

Members of Parliament presumably saw things similarly. In 1993 the
Courts and Legal Services Act 1990 was amended to establish "no win,
no fee." Under this law clients could elect to pay lawyers double fees if
their claims succeeded and nothing if they failed.[19] The expansion of this
arrangement after a limited initial trial period enabled people who were

too poor to cover the legal costs themselves and not poor enough to qualify for legal aid to sue without up-front expenses.[20] Then, with the stated objective of excluding from litigation cases deemed unlikely to succeed, the handling of Legal Aid clinical negligence cases was closed to all but specialist firms in 1999. The new rules both reduced the number of cases filed and increased the proportion of those filed that succeeded.[21]

Should the United States limit health care spending, geographical diversity and the independence of states in defining malpractice would pose difficult analytical, political, and ethical issues different from those that have arisen in Great Britain (see chapter 8).

Political and Social Responses to Resource Constraints

The British press of the early 1980s contained only two reports addressing palpable inadequacies in medical care. One quoted a nephrologist who was impatient at having "to tell lies to older patients, partly to make the patients more comfortable and partly to make ourselves more comfortable. . . . We are getting fed up with telling lies."[22] The other report complained about underfunding of "bone marrow transplants, leading apparently to the deaths of many children who could have been saved if more cash were available for transplant programmes."[23] This near silence has given way to routine discussion of health care inadequacies. Newspaper exposés report waiting lists, lack of equipment, and other service inadequacies. Daily television reports tell of superior care on offer in other nations of the European community. It seems beyond doubt that an avalanche of press and television reports and congressional hearings about services denied and hardships endured would quickly follow the introduction of spending limits in the United States.

Summary

The patterns of behavior described in this chapter are the natural responses of patients and providers to a system of medical care characterized by insufficient resources to satisfy patients' demands. British history, politics, social relations, and national psychology powerfully influence those responses. Even so, growing British protests against limits have come increasingly to resemble what would likely occur in the United States. The operative question in the United States would not be how to mobilize people to assert their wants and needs, but whether resistance would prevent such controls from ever coming into being or, if established, from being enforced.

British experience suggests certain generalizations about which sorts of medical care would be curtailed most by budget limits. First, services that depend on dedicated capital equipment and highly specialized staff would be cut more than services that can be provided by regular hospital personnel and supplies. A lack of inputs critical to a particular form of care would confront physicians with a fait accompli. Second, arcane services for which the need is not readily understood by patients will be curtailed more than will services for which the need is clear and inescapable. Third, constraints will reduce services that claim a large or growing share of the health budget proportionately more than they do those that claim a small share.

In addition, physicians and patients would develop ways to make life more tolerable under budget constraints. In Britain physicians often adjust indications for treatment to align demand with resource availability. This kind of rationalization preserves as much as possible the feeling that all care of value is being provided.

The willingness of most British patients to accept their doctor's word, once taken for granted by British providers, is gradually beginning to give way to a new assertiveness. Though seemingly not as insistent as their U.S. counterparts, British patients of today are far more likely to protest denial of care than were those of past generations. Safety valves have always allowed persistent patients to circumvent limits imposed by the National Health Service. Patients can pay to see consultants, to gain access to a pay bed in an NHS hospital, or to secure admission in a private facility. In special cases they may travel to the continent for care. But, increasingly, patients are complaining about the NHS, and the political system is responding. The Blair government has raised health care funding faster than at any time in NHS history and has promised to keep health budgets rising. As always, patients who are denied care can try to use friends or relatives to gain access to care or present themselves directly to a specialized unit where it is hard for the physician in charge to turn them away. To an increasing extent, patients have begun to turn to the British legal system to secure redress for care they deem inadequate. Most such litigation arises from medical errors avoidable even in a budget-constrained system, but it is often hard to draw a bright line between simple error and care denied because of resource scarcity. These behaviors, which have changed in degree but not in kind over the past two decades, are consistent with both intuition and common sense.

Whether these behaviors and the ways they have changed have important implications for Americans depends on the likelihood that the United States would adopt and sustain effective budget controls and on the form such controls might take. The next and final chapter examines this critical question.

CHAPTER EIGHT

Rationing Health Care in the United States

Many Americans find unthinkable the idea that the United States might one day ration medical care. The fact that millions are entirely uninsured or lack adequate coverage is widely accepted, if regretted. However, in a strange exercise in mental compartmentalization, limits on care for those with good health insurance or enough money to pay seem strange and unthinkable. Yet continuation of past rates of growth in health care spending portend unprecedented government deficits, rising numbers of uninsured, and narrowed capacity of U.S. workers to enjoy increases in other forms of consumption.[1]

To be sure, future increases in health care spending promise huge *net* benefits. But they also threaten much increased spending on care worth less than it costs. The glorious promise of modern medicine thereby raises the stakes on eliminating low-benefit care. Limiting low-benefit care can help ensure the affordability of the magnificent range of life-extending, pain-relieving, aging-retarding advances spawned by biomedical research. Rather than being seen as an un-American and gruesome betrayal of an unlimited commitment to life, health care rationing should be recognized as essential to realizing the promise of tomorrow's medicine at an affordable price.

For many, "rationing" is a four-letter word. They seem to have in mind the mindless denial of care, whether or not it is worth what it costs. Such rationing deserves all of the scorn heaped on it. But intelligent rationing, informed by solid research on the medical results of various procedures and people's evaluations of those results, will increase social welfare. And, if rationing averts misconceived efforts to lower health care spending for vulnerable populations or to reduce spending on medical research, it can improve overall health care as well.

Cost Growth—Past and Future

The realization that rising health care spending is problematic is not new. More than three decades ago the administration of Richard Nixon instituted direct price controls on hospitals. Then the administration of Jimmy Carter tried unsuccessfully to persuade Congress to regulate hospital costs. The growth of health care spending abated during the 1990s. Employers intensified their bargaining with hospitals and other providers. Managed care spread throughout the nation. Medicare instituted prospective payment, first for hospitals and later for other providers. Medicare also established fee schedules for physicians and other services.[2] Congress slowed the annual increase in Medicare payments to hospitals and physicians.[3] States negotiated lower Medicaid payments. Criminal and civil prosecution punished overbilling by Medicare providers. These measures helped slow the growth of per capita health care spending to barely more than the growth of per capita income, lulling some observers into believing that the threat of endless health care inflation had ended.[4]

This optimism was misplaced. The slowdown of the 1990s, it now seems clear, largely reflected one-time savings. Health care cost inflation accelerated after 2000. Recent breakthroughs in molecular biology and information technology suggest that the pace of advances in medical technology will not slow and may accelerate.[5] Population aging continues relentlessly. Only drastic cuts in Medicare and Medicaid that would undermine the basic objectives of these programs can prevent government-financed health care spending from greatly outpacing growth of GDP.

Past forecast errors should teach forecasters humility. ("Give a number or a date, but never both," a well-known Scottish economist once advised.) But past errors do not nullify the powerful forces driving health care spending. For four decades growth in health care spending has exceeded income growth by an average of 2.5 percentage points a year. Tables 8-1 and 8-2 show that if these trends continue health care spending will dominate government budgets and claim one-third or more of

Table 8-1. *Medicare and Medicaid Expenditures as Percent of GDP and the Federal Budget, Selected Years*

| | Growth of health care spending exceeds growth of income by | | | |
| | 2.5 percentage points | | 1 percentage point | |
Year	GDP[a]	Federal outlays[b]	GDP[a]	Federal outlays[b]
2005	4.2	19.6	4.2	19.6
2010	5.3	23.2	4.8	22.5
2020	7.8	28.9	6.5	27.7
2030	11.5	33.6	8.4	30.8
2040	16.1	36.1	10.1	32.2

Sources: Figures for 2005 are estimates taken from Congressional Budget Office (CBO), *The Budget and Economic Outlook: Fiscal Years 2006 to 2015* (January 2005). Figures for subsequent years are projections from CBO, *The Long-Term Budget Outlook* (December 2003).

a. National outlays on Medicaid as a share of GDP include spending by state and local governments, set at two-thirds of federal outlays.

b. Federal outlays net out premium payments because they are not a share of federal costs. GDP shares are based on the gross cost of services paid in full or in part by Medicare and Medicaid.

GDP. Even if it exceeds income growth by only one percentage point a year, growth of health care spending will squeeze government budgets and private incomes.

Without major intervention there is no reason to expect this 2.5 percentage point gap between growth of incomes and health care spending to narrow. The challenge is clear. Americans will either spend ever more on low-benefit health care, or they will have to ration care for some or all of those who are insured.

Alternatives to Rationing—Realistic Prospects or Blind Alleys?

Numerous "solutions" have been proposed to avoid rationing care for the well insured. These include managed care, bulk buying by providers, computerization, a shift to prepaid group practice, selective contracting with doctors and hospitals who provide high-quality care at low cost, eliminating wasteful care—such as defensive medicine allegedly induced by the threat of malpractice litigation—and increased cost sharing.

Table 8-2. *Total Health Care Spending as Percent of GDP, Alternative Growth Rates for Health Care Spending, Selected Years*

	Growth of health care spending exceeds growth of GDP by	
Year	2.5 percentage points	1 percentage point
2005	15.6[a]	15.6[a]
2010	17.3[a]	17.3[a]
2020	21.6	19.8
2030	27.6	21.9
2040	35.2	24.1

Sources: Except as noted, data are from Henry J. Aaron and Jack Meyer, "Health," in *Restoring Fiscal Sanity: Meeting the Long Run Challenge,* edited by Alice Rivlin and Isabel Sawhill (Brookings, 2005).

a. Stephen Heffler and others, "U.S. Health Spending Projections for 2004–2014," *Health Affairs* (content.healthaffairs.org/cgi/content/abstract/hlthaff.w5.74 [February 23, 2005]); Congressional Budget Office, "The Long-Term Budget Outlook, December 2003" (www.cbo.gov/showdoc.cfm?index=4916&sequence=0 [July 2005]).

Is Eliminating "Waste" the Answer?

Such measures as bulk buying and electronic billing and record keeping can achieve genuine one-time savings. They may even improve the quality of care. But they will not block the cost pressures that make consideration of rationing inescapable. And in some cases—the institution of electronic billing or computerization of medical records, for example—they will raise spending in the near term.[6]

Much standard medical care provides no demonstrable benefit. Evaluations of medical records indicate that a quarter or more of certain procedures should not have been prescribed.[7] As much as a quarter of Medicare spending seems to contribute nothing to survival.[8] Some observers have concluded from these studies that simply eliminating waste can keep Medicare solvent, dramatically slow growth of total health care spending, and avoid the pain of rationing.

This hope is almost certainly illusory. The fact that the most recent studies report as much "waste" as did studies released two decades ago suggests that even if such waste can be curbed, the process will take a very long time. Nor is such "unnecessary" care confined to the high-spending United States. Over 20 percent of hospital stays in the University Hospital of Maastricht in the Netherlands were found to be inappropriate.[9] Research from Germany reported that 28 percent of surgical hospital days and one-third of medical hospital days were inappropriate.[10] A program to reduce inappropriate hospital stays at one Barcelona hospital lowered the proportion of such stays from 36 percent to 28 percent. But after the program ended, the proportion of inappropriate stays returned to 33 percent.[11] Even in resource-limited Great Britain 35 percent of referrals from primary to secondary care were found to be inappropriate.[12]

Why is elimination of waste so difficult, slow, and prone to backsliding? To dislodge suboptimal practices requires difficult, controversial, and time-consuming studies. Even when research establishing the efficacy of particular interventions is available, success in persuading all physicians to apply the practice has proved spotty. Eliminating waste will also require a change in how new physicians are trained and in how currently active physicians practice. These changes take time. Meanwhile, technological advance and population aging will continue unabated.

Finally, and most important, a growing body of research shows that underprovision of health care is also a serious problem in the United States. More patients fail to receive medically indicated care than are given unnecessary or inappropriate care. Although 20 percent of patients received unnecessary or "contraindicated" chronic care, and 30 percent received contraindicated acute care, 30 percent of patients did not receive recommended acute care, 40 percent did not receive recommended chronic care, and 50 percent did not receive recommended preventive care.[13] Furthermore, overuse, which is documented in patients' records, is more likely to be identified than underuse, which must be inferred.[14]

A successful campaign to target health care more accurately would improve the quality of health care per dollar spent, but whether it would lower or raise spending is far from clear.

Is Prepaid Health Insurance the Answer?

Advocates of prepaid medical care have long asserted that health maintenance organizations (HMOs) hold the answer to slowing the growth of medical costs. HMOs hospitalize patients less often and hold outlays below those of fee-for-service providers.[15] Critics counter that HMOs undertreat. Advocates respond that although HMOs use a different mix of outpatient and inpatient care, the care is as good on the average as that of other health plans.

HMOs cannot promise a sustained slow-down in the growth of health care spending unless the gap between their costs and those of conventional insurance widens. In fact, the gap has been constant. Furthermore, prepaid plans of all kinds, including many with looser spending controls than standard HMOs, cover only about 36 percent of all insured Americans, and membership in traditional HMOs has not increased recently.[16] Patients have resisted the limits HMOS impose and insist on the right to receive care outside the closed panels of physicians and other providers that HMOs typically employ. HMOs may be slower to introduce certain new technologies and manage with less of them, but they are subject to the same technological forces affecting other providers.[17] Some applications of new technologies will be highly beneficial; others will be of little or no value. To summarize: even if prepaid plans came to cover everyone—a prospect that seems remote—long-term cost containment would still require that hard choices be made about who gets what kind of care.

Although prepaid health plans cannot eliminate the need to confront rationing's dilemma, they may well help the nation to deal with it. The key is capitation: the specification of a sum that covers all care provided in a given prospective period.[18] Prepaid plans can accommodate safety valves for patients seeking additional care. For example, the plan may provide limited coverage for patients to buy care outside the system at additional cost. Prepaid plans create entities that lend themselves to regulatory control—from enrollees or from public authorities. Thus prepaid plans cannot avoid rationing as some of their advocates claim, but they may offer a way to implement it.

Are Medicare-Type Controls the Answer?

The elaborate set of administered prices for individual episodes of care employed by traditional Medicare has clearly failed to rein in health care spending.[19] The most fundamental problem with event-based prepayment based on administered prices is that such systems, by design, control prices, not quantities. They do nothing to limit low-benefit services, such as the marginal outpatient MRI scan or dialysis on the terminally ill patient, whose death is negligibly delayed and whose suffering may be protracted.

Prepayment based on capitation—a flat fee per patient for a fixed period—reverses quantity incentives so that providers have no direct financial gain from providing added services. Fixed budgets have the same effect. Traditional HMOs use the former device; the British National Health Service uses the latter. Neither approach is immune to daunting regulatory problems. Neither avoids the need, as technology advances, to ration in order to achieve sustained reductions in the growth of health care spending. But both provide a framework for debate about how much rationing is socially optimal. The excessive incentives to increase quantity under fee-for-service and the entire absence of such incentives under fixed budgets or capitation suggest that a blended system of capitation together with modest payments for additional services may be a superior option.[20]

Implementing Limits

The same forces drive health care spending everywhere: income, the extent of insurance or other third-party payment arrangements, the age distribution of the population, technological progress, and public regulation.

Over the past half century, every developed nation has in some way protected all or nearly all patients from most or all of the cost of care when sick. Even in the United States, which lags in this regard, approximately 85 percent of the population is insured publicly or privately. U.S. regulation of health care spending differs markedly from that of every other developed nation as well. In other nations the government or private entities representing sizable fractions of the population limit health care spending through negotiating power or legislation. The U.S. system is, in fact, bereft of any effective ways to discourage well-insured patients from seeking care that generates any benefit, however small. It is highly fragmented, with numerous public and private buyers and a huge number of disconnected sellers of health care.

Such a system has many appealing features. It easily caters to diverse local preferences. One size need not fit all. U.S. health care is relatively free of bottlenecks, so that waiting lists and waiting times are rarely long. But a fragmented system, such as that of the United States, has serious drawbacks as well. No agent has enough power to override the incentives for well-insured patients to demand more health care than is socially optimal. The weakness of financial limits undercuts incentives for cost-reducing research (see Victor Fuchs and Alan Garber's metaphorical example presented in chapter 1). Administrative costs are staggeringly high.[21]

If the United States is ever to control the growth of health care costs and spending, major changes in the way health care is financed or organized must occur. One option is to tighten eligibility criteria for public programs. In both public and private plans, the range of services covered could be narrowed, or cost sharing could be increased.

How far such measures can or should be extended is unclear, however. The largest public programs cover populations with few economic resources—the poor and disabled through Medicaid, and the elderly and disabled through Medicare. Medicaid eligibility is conditioned on a lack of income and assets. If coverage is narrowed, those served would have few options other than to go without care. Only 12 percent of Medicare enrollees have incomes in excess of $50,000 a year. The scope for increased cost sharing in public programs is therefore quite limited without creating hardships for people of quite modest means. Very large increases in the age of eligibility would be necessary to make a major dent in Medicare outlays. To hold growth of per capita Medicare spending to per capita income growth, the age of eligibility would have to be increased to seventy-nine by 2030 and eighty-three by 2040, or the proportion of personal health care spending covered by Medicare would have to be halved by 2030 and cut by nearly two-thirds by 2040.[22]

In the private sector, a trend toward narrowed benefit packages and increased cost sharing is clearly apparent. Employers are raising premiums, deductibles and other copayments, narrowing benefit packages, or dropping sponsorship of health plans altogether. As a result employees increasingly decline coverage for themselves or their dependents. As health care cost inflation continues, experts expect coverage to narrow still further.[23] If they are right, then coverage for the majority with moderate incomes will be constrained, while people with higher incomes will retain the capacity to buy more complete insurance coverage or to pay directly for care when it is needed. This development would mean the emergence of highly differentiated standards of care based on income and wealth. Such differentiation is normal with respect to most commodities, but it is contrary to widely held values on the desirability of relatively equal access to a service as central as health care is to life and well-being. In terms relevant to this book, it would sustain low-benefit care for those with the means to pay for it, while increasingly narrowing access, perhaps even to high-benefit care, for those without the financial resources.

The natural way to avoid such an outcome would be to extend coverage to essentially all Americans and to accept regulatory limits on total health care spending by all. What this means is that universal health insurance coverage is desirable not only for the reasons traditionally emphasized—that it would improve financial access to health care—but also because it is a precondition for reducing the use of low-benefit care by all. It also means that the United States should invest far more than it now does in careful evaluation of the efficacy of medical procedures so that decisions can be based on better information than is now available about what works and what does not.

Analysts have outlined a variety of ways to achieve near-universal coverage. Individuals could be mandated to show that they and their families have health insurance, backed up by direct subsidies or tax breaks for those who cannot afford the premiums. Employers could be required to sponsor and pay for part of the cost of health insurance for employees and their families. A centralized government-managed health insurance plan could be established to replace or supplement current coverage.

Each of these approaches has identifiable strengths and weaknesses. None is new. None has come close to achieving majority support at the national level. To break this logjam, the federal government could provide financial support to states, acting alone or in groups, that made progress in reducing the numbers of uninsured. Each state could use whatever method its residents found congenial.[24] But universal coverage, by one means or another, is a prerequisite for instituting limits that would create incentives to equitably reduce the prevalence of low-benefit care. A system in which 45 million people are without any health insurance at all and millions of others are poorly insured remains tolerable only because the uninsured have access to considerable amounts of health care, particularly during serious illness, that is supported through a complex web of cross-subsidies—costs shifted to the insured and paid by them. Efforts to limit spending by the well-insured will inevitably undercut their willingness to tolerate these cross-subsidies.

Furthermore, a system as fragmented as that in the United States provides no mechanism for effectively limiting aggregate spending. The device that is used to ensure near-universal coverage would also serve as the lever for controlling expenditures. The lever could be tax incentives, direct regulation, or payments through public programs. In all cases, however, the wide diversity of patient preferences, medical practice patterns, and local conditions in a country as large and diverse as the United States would make it desireable for individual patients, their health care providers, and local organizations to retain control over the allocation of available funds.

The Challenges of Health Care Rationing

The advent of rationing will force the nation to confront new and unfamiliar problems. With weak limits, few changes in actual medical practice might be observed. At some point, however, decisions would have to be made on what services should be curtailed and how to manage a system in which not everyone who stands to benefit from care can be treated. Although such decisions should reflect the shape of the benefit curve for each form of treatment, as indicated in chapter 6, such data are lacking for most therapies. So is good information on personal valuations of medical outcomes.[25] Even with more complete information than now exists, legitimation of the resulting decisions would be formidably difficult.

The United States would face issues similar to those Britain has confronted, except that the United States would start from a much higher base. Although objective sacrifices would be less severe than those in Britain, they would likely be perceived as more painful because insured Americans have never experienced the denial of services long familiar to the British.

As constraints increased, the effects on patient care would intensify. The introduction of expensive new treatments would likely be slowed until, or even after, effectiveness is clearly demonstrated. Even if expenditures on patients considered to have a high probability of survival were unconstrained, the projected budget pressures from increases in Medicare and Medicaid spending would likely cause U.S. treatment of the terminally ill to resemble practice in Britain, where scarcity of intensive care beds and other specialized technologies limit aggressive care.

Such changes would occur because resource limits would create a new reality. Even now, U.S. doctors realize that aggressive treatment of many terminally ill patients is often pointless. They continue treatment nonetheless, sometimes because the patient's family insists, sometimes because they fear malpractice suits, and sometimes because courts intervene. Courts now routinely apply absolutist standards. Thus failure to provide care that promises even small medical benefits is considered malpractice. The economic effect of providing all beneficial care is widely diffused—it simply raises someone's taxes or premiums. With limited resources, the effects would be sharply focused—services used to keep alive a comatose or impaired terminally ill patient for a few days or weeks would be unavailable to spare a nonterminally ill patient death, disability, and pain. Battlefield physicians with insufficient resources to care for everyone have long understood and accepted that time and medication should be used to help those who stand to benefit most. The same ethic will emerge under resource constraints.

Limitations on New Therapies

British experience suggests that budget limits slow but do not prevent the introduction of new therapies. Normally the use of new procedures grows with time as techniques are perfected and additional applications are unearthed. Budget limits would slow this process. Use of new technologies would be lower for many more years than in a system without constraints. It is likely that therapies already in use when limits are imposed will be affected less than new therapies. Preventing new habits from being formed is easier than breaking old ones.

Research indicates that basic science responds to external economic incentives as well as to the internal dynamics of scientific discovery. Thus budget limits are likely both to reduce and to redirect private research spending. A slowdown in the application of discoveries in molecular biology, for example, could delay cures for major causes of death and disability. A redirection of science to less costly ways of achieving given medical outcomes would likely occur quite slowly but might eventually produce sizable savings. The potential impact on the pace and direction of scientific development is perhaps the most important and least predictable effect of budget limits.

Total Cost of New Technology

The total cost of a new technology will also influence how rapidly it is introduced and how widely it is made available.[26] Limited budgets in the United States would require U.S. health care providers to decide explicitly whether investments in new technology are justified, just as their British counterparts have been forced to do. The answer could well be "yes" if intervention provides patients with years of high-quality life. The answer would almost certainly be "no" if such large investments extend life only briefly or left the patient in pain and immobilized.

Waiting Lists

Reducing hospital admissions usually saves money. Curtailing discretionary hospitalizations directly lowers admissions. If waiting lists develop, they lower admissions indirectly: some people decide not to get in the queue in the first place, others improve while waiting, and some die. Still another way to lower admissions is to close treatment facilities, thereby increasing patients' average travel time and cost and lowering demand.

All of these approaches are controversial. Community residents fight to keep hospitals open. Lengthy waiting lists provoke controversy. Americans are unaccustomed to waiting and would protest vigorously if they had to do so. Physicians and other providers, especially those paid on a fee-for-service basis, might join patients in protesting waiting lists. And where patients and physicians sound the alarm about delays in care, investigative reporters, congressional hearings, and political intervention would not be far behind. Mute acceptance of lengthy queues for elective surgery by U.S. patients is hard to imagine. If no private-sector safety valves exists for those who are unwilling to wait and have the means to pay, pressure to relax regulations will become irresistible long before queues became as long they have been in Britain.

Response of Physicians

British experience suggests that budget limits would gradually cause accepted standards of practice to change, despite the contrary incentives of fee-for-service medicine. "Good" medicine would call for fewer tests. U.S. physicians might begin to tell themselves, as their British counterparts do, that ultrasound often is an adequate, if not optimal, alternative to CT or MRI scans, particularly in nonemergency cases. Less surgery and less costly drugs would come to be regarded as "standard" when the medical advantage of expensive over inexpensive therapies is small. In short, U.S. doctors would begin to build into their own norms of good practice a sense of the relation between the costs and benefits of care. They would be led to weigh not only the medical aspects of diagnosis and treatment but also the peculiar circumstances of each patient: age, underlying health, family responsibilities, and chance of recovering enough to resume a normal life.

This process would make obsolete the view, once held by many American doctors, that weighing costs in deciding what actions to take on behalf of patients is not only unprofessional, but downright immoral. Physicians today still recognize their personal responsibility to act as their patients' agents. But most already understand that resources are not unlimited and that trade-offs are a legitimate subject for national debate. Although U.S. physicians would likely continue to act as their patients' agents, spending limits would cause them, like their British counterparts, to redefine "appropriate" care.

British experience indicates that the care most easily denied is that requiring costly capital goods or specially trained staff. If the authorities do not invest in the capital goods or hire the staff, the services cannot be provided. Providers are placed in the position of simply doing all they can in the time available. Staff may be overworked and possibly grumpy. But they will not be guilt-ridden or conflicted by the need to deny care they had the power to give. External constraints spare providers the psychologically insupportable burden of *deciding* to withhold care. A bureaucrat, antiseptically removed from confrontation with the sick and their families, performs that odious task by making a budget decision. Providers have the job of allocating existing capacity to the patients who will benefit most from it. They also have the mixed blessing of using their spare time and energy to fight for more. No British doctors interviewed for this book said that cost dictated care for particular patients when capital-intensive activity was considered. Capacity limits, resulting from earlier decisions on investment and staffing, forced them to make choices. Because external constraints facilitate saying "no," capital-intensive services and those requiring large numbers of specially trained personnel would likely be primary targets for holding down expenditures. The use of negotiated, fixed-fee, or capitated payments for specialist providers who handle particular classes of care—treatment of cancer, diabetes, or established coronary disease, for example—is likely to spread. Such contracts effectively control spending while shifting decisions about modes of care to others. They may also yield improved care through specialization.

Services that do not require dedicated capital equipment or specially trained providers are hard but not impossible to ration. In HMOs plan managers can supervise how salaried physicians use their time and prescribe various procedures. In health plans paying physicians on a fee-for-service basis, fees can be set to discourage particular modes of care. Pharmaceutical benefits managers can use copayments and formularies to encourage use of generic or inexpensive drugs as alternatives to costly patented drugs.

Nonetheless, aggressive doctors can and do lay claim to extra resources by incremental steps. British nephrologists pushed home dialysis to circumvent limits on hospital-based dialysis. Limiting in-hospital use of drugs, blood, and other expendable supplies by monitoring day-to-day clinical decisions would be almost impossible. Because such micromanagement is impracticable, physicians could be constrained only if their use of resources was so excessive that, as in Britain, their colleagues forced a change in behavior.

Response of Patients

U.S. patients have come to expect all medical services from which they might benefit. They are likely to fight service cuts more aggressively than have the British, and their opportunity to do so would be incomparably greater. Most U.S. patients may see any general practitioner or specialist with whom they can secure an appointment. The fee-for-service system encourages most physicians to give them one. Thus, the scope for patients to cajole, browbeat, or essentially bribe doctors to provide "full" care is vast. Consequently, the relative advantage of aggressive patients with money in securing superior care would probably increase in a resource-limited system.

Care outside the System

Many patients who face limits on health care spending would seek care outside the regulated system. A central regulatory and political question for any system of controls is whether and on what terms to authorize care outside the controls. Such care may be prohibited, as it was in Canada, until a court decision declared the bar unconstitutional.[27] Or it may be permitted, but made costly to patients. How large that additional cost should be is as critical an issue as the stringency of controls.

The provision of care outside a cost-controlled system can be discouraged by such traditional regulatory instruments as the tax system, licensing, and limits on reimbursement through public programs or private insurance. Each approach would create distinct political, administrative, and economic problems.[28] If care outside the controlled system were precluded, some patients might go to Canada or elsewhere, where entrepreneurs could be expected to extend the services already offered abroad. The affluent would be the principal "importers" of foreign health care, much as the wealthy from poor countries now seek health care in the United States and elsewhere. Just as the well-to-do can buy superior education for their children in private schools, they are likely to be the principal users of medical care safety valves to buy more or better health care, contributing to the development of two-class health care, with a higher standard for those with the means to "buy out" of constraints.

Charity

Providers may try to escape budget limits by seeking charity. U.S. hospitals now solicit individual and foundation philanthropy. Incentives to promote such giving would increase with the restrictiveness of expenditure constraints.[29] Such gifts would not merely express charitable impulses. They would become a safety valve permitting individuals or communities to buy medical services the budget does not support.

Whatever the motivation for such gifts, the authorities must decide what to do about them. Spending controls that encompass all services, however financed, would strongly discourage charitable contributions because gifts would merely supplant other payments. Alternatively, charitable gifts could be permitted, or even encouraged, precisely because they relax spending constraints. Indeed, health planners might strategically shortchange precisely those services or facilities that potential donors could be expected to support. Policies that permit exit from the controlled system and encourage charitable giving may help sustain tight formal budget limits even as they boost outlays. Policies that discourage exit and charitable giving will increase the political resistance to budget limits because vocal and influential groups will protest constraints on their right to enhance availability of health care services.

Litigation

Spending limits that force rationing would raise new and troubling problems for medical liability litigation. Historically the courts have almost always found health care providers nonculpable if they complied with "customary standards of medical practice."[30] This rule is coherent and enforceable if a health care system provides all beneficial care. It is coherent also in a budget-limited system if some central body establishes uniform standards of treatment. It is not coherent if separate elements of the health care system are free to use limited resources in different ways.

If spending limits deny some patients beneficial care, some who are denied care will suffer adverse outcomes and sue. They will point to standards of practice in other areas where the care they were denied is actually given. Would courts in city X, where, say, MRIs come to be regarded as inappropriate for low back pain but essential for diagnosing arthritic knees, sustain such practices if in city Y physicians have reverse priorities? Absent a degree of centralized decisionmaking that is unthinkable in the United States, disparate uses of limited resources are inescapable. Therapies unavailable in one place might be plentiful elsewhere. Patients denied a service available at one institution would allege that arbitrary decisions had violated their right to equal protection under the law. Procedures for allocating budgets would be challenged on similar grounds. What would be judged "customary practice"? What would the courts do?

Such litigation could threaten the sustainability of expenditure controls unless national criteria for judging medical negligence emerged. The redefinition of negligence would be slow and contentious. Litigation over the myriad medical decisions appealable under current law could both choke the courts and paralyze medical practice. This risk would increase the urgency of shifting most disputes regarding alleged malpractice from the courts to a nonadversarial venue.

Political Pressure

As experience amply shows, patients denied beneficial care will be grist for exposés and congressional hearings. Patients or relatives of patients denied care will write their elected representatives who will recognize the wide appeal of heartrending stories. Television cameras will carry congressional hearings to millions of viewers. Legislative and executive staff will bring pressure to bear on hospitals or insurance plans. Pressure from constituents might cause Congress to except "just this one" service from the limits. Such piecemeal exceptions would weaken and could destroy controls and would undoubtedly complicate administration.

These pressures are not hypothetical. States use their power to regulate insurance to require that approved plans include coverage of many specific services. Congress has mandated that specific services must be provided to Medicare enrollees. It enacted special legislation requiring the courts to reconsider whether the feeding tube of a woman in a persistent vegetative state should be reinserted despite repeated prior rulings that its removal was medically justified. These examples do not suggest that efforts to control spending growth are ill advised. But they do presage similar responses to new and expensive technologies.

Conclusions

All developed nations have devised institutions to insulate patients from having to weigh costs and benefits when ill and to spare them financial ruination from costly treatment. None relies to a significant degree on cost sharing to limit spending because all understand that sufficient cost sharing to limit spending growth would expose patients to the very financial risks from which insurance is intended to protect them. The particular mechanisms of control differ from country to country. To hold down costs, all developed nations other than the United States have fashioned administrative controls to limit spending.

Modern medicine possesses a large and growing armory of increasingly costly weapons for dealing with illness. It produces great benefits for some. It also produces small benefits relative to cost for others. The United States will soon be forced to think about whether to join other nations in finding ways to encourage patients and providers to humanely weigh the benefits and costs of medical care.

The British simply legislate how much the health care system can spend. Little support exists in the United States for that approach. But the United States faces staggering increases in health care spending, both private and public. Patients with adequate incomes are likely to face steadily rising out-of-pocket payments levied to hold down health care spending. But most health care is consumed during serious illnesses when insurance "stop-loss" provisions shield patients from all costs of care. Continued growth of health care expenditures will therefore force Americans to consider heretofore unthinkable ways to limit spending. The federal government, at various times, has tried to hold down costs by limiting purchases of equipment and controlling the number of hospital beds. These programs enjoyed few successes. For the most part, they have vanished. Various presidents proposed federal limits on hospital spending. Congress authorized, and administrators gradually introduced, fixed prospective payment for most Medicare services. Private health plans have adopted a wide range of administrative measures, subsumed under the name "managed care," to slow growth of spending but without sustained effect.

In the future, old ways of slowing the growth of health care spending will return, and new methods will be tried. The fundamental conflict between a fee-for-service system of reimbursing physicians and efforts to limit health care spending is inescapable. New policies will have to be developed regarding safety valves, medical negligence, and the introduction of new technologies—policies that current ways of providing medical care do not require.

No one can anticipate in exactly what way or how vigorously the United States will try to hold down health care spending. Many forces will be arrayed against the implementation and enforcement of limits that ration care; that cut into incomes of doctors, nurses, and other staff; or that significantly curtail sales by drug companies, equipment manufacturers, and other suppliers. It would be possible, but formidably expensive, for the United States simply to "let 'er rip" and pay for all the care that well-insured patients seek and providers supply. It is possible that at each point, the steps needed to limit spending growth may seem less appealing than paying just a bit more for health care than last year. But this course implies enormous tax increases, considerable loss of social welfare, and the allocation of a growing proportion of, and eventually all, increases in private worker compensation to health care. It would imply lower national economic welfare and poorer health for the nation as a whole than will be possible if we adopt sensible measures to squeeze out care that costs more than it is worth.

The choices are clear. We can simply pay the enormous bill for all beneficial medical care whatever the cost. Or we can ration. If we follow the second course, we must begin by extending health care to essentially all Americans. We shall then have to confront a long list of hard decisions, on few of which has discussion even begun. Rationing will inevitably be controversial and difficult to implement, but like bitter but efficacious medicine, it can be good for our nation's health.

Frequency
of Surgery

In the late 1970s, the British did three-fourths to four-fifths as many total hip replacements and nearly as much orthopedic surgery of all kinds as Americans did.[1] A higher proportion of operations performed by the British were operations short of hip replacement, possibly in connection with broken hips of elderly people.[2] That difference between the rate of hip operations performed in the United States and in Great Britain has narrowed or vanished. The British now do an estimated 94 to 100 percent as many total hip replacements as the Americans do.

The data underlying this conclusion are far from ideal. One overarching problem concerns which types of patients are included:

—every patient who received hip operations, whether as inpatients or in emergency departments;

—only patients who received *inpatient* operations, whether admitted directly or through emergency wards; or

—only patients admitted directly to inpatient wards, excluding emergency admissions altogether. Recent British data are available for the latter two groups only. Recent U.S. data are readily available only for the second.

U.S. Data

Since the late 1980s, the primary source of data on the frequency of hip operations performed in U.S. hospitals has been the Healthcare Cost and

Table A-1. *Hip Replacements Performed in the United States, 1979 and 2000*

Units as indicated

Procedure	1979	2000	Percent increase
Total hip replacement			
Number performed	71,700	198,873	177
Rate per million	313	707	126
Rate per million age 60+	2,012	4,342	116
Partial hip replacement			
Number performed	73,300	109,182	49
Rate per million	324	388	20
Rate per million age 60+	2,057	2,284	16
All hip replacements			
Number performed	145,000	308,055	112
Rate per million	637	1,095	71
Rate per million age 60+	4,069	6,727	65

Sources: For the 1979 numbers, see Henry J. Aaron and William B. Schwartz, *The Painful Prescription: Rationing Hospital Care* (Brookings, 1984), p. 137; for 2000 data, see Agency for Healthcare Research and Quality, "Healthcare Cost Utilization Project (HCUP)" (www.ahrq.gov/data/hcup/hcupstat.htm [July 2005]).

Utilization Project (HCUP) database, maintained by the Agency for Healthcare Research and Quality. The data are broken down under three headings: total hip replacement, partial hip replacement, and revision hip replacement. These procedures were not tabulated separately in the 1970s.[3]

While the specific classifications are not directly comparable between the 1970s and today, it is reasonable to compare the sum of the various categories between years. Table A-1 does just this. It shows that more hip operations are performed today than two decades ago, both in absolute and relative terms. In 1979 about 637 people per million received hip replacements of all kinds in the United States, compared to 1,095 per million in 2000, an increase of over 70 percent.[4]

Given that revision procedures are classified separately in the recent data, gauging shifts in frequency of total hip replacements since 1979, rather than all hip operations combined, requires estimation. According to the HCUP data, 165,065 primary (nonrevision) hip replacements were performed in 2000. According to another source, about 83 percent of all total hip replacements performed on Medicare patients in 1997 were primary replacements and 17 percent were revisions.[5] If these proportions apply also to non-Medicare patients and have remained constant since 1997, one can estimate that nearly 198,000 total hip replacements were performed in 2000, significantly more than the 71,700 performed in 1979.[6] The actual total is probably somewhat smaller as Medicare patients are older and therefore more likely to have revisions than non-Medicare patients.[7] As table A-1 shows, the per capita increase in hip replacement procedures performed since the late 1970s is primarily due to increases in total hip replacements rather than partial implants.

British Data

Ambiguous data on hip replacements performed in Britain in the late 1970s pose problems for gauging trends in procedures performed since that time. Since the late 1980s, the main source of data on the frequency of various procedures performed in NHS hospitals in England has been the Department of Health's Hospital Episode Statistics (HES). Table A-2 shows the headings under which the earlier data were collected and how they compare to headings used for HES data. Both sets of data tabulate "total hip replacements." But the headings for hip operations less extensive than total replacement are not strictly comparable. As the second and third rows of table A-2 show, the categories used to classify procedures in the earlier data were ambiguous and broader than those used for the recent data. It is possible, however, to ascertain the number of operations performed in connection with "fractured neck of femur," which is comparable to recent statistics. So despite the ambiguity of the original British data, one can gauge shifts in the frequency of total hip replacement as well as for one specific category of partial replacements.

Table A-3 shows the results of this exercise. Two points are worth noting. First, the British Department of Health, along with most other government departments, has experienced significant devolution. As a result, health statistics are no longer collected at the national level. So while the earlier statistics capture procedures performed in England and Wales combined, recent statistics capture only procedures carried out in England. When examining trends, therefore, it is more accurate to compare population-adjusted rates than absolute numbers of operations. Second, as noted above, it is unclear whether the 1977 data dealt with emergency

Table A-2. *Comparability of British Data, 1977 and 2000*[a]

Units as indicated

1977		2000		
Procedure heading	*Number performed*	*HES procedure heading*	*Number performed*	*Comment*
"Arthroplasty associated with osteoarthritis, namely total hip replacement"	14,200	Total prosthetic replacement of hip joint	41,546	Comparable
"Arthroplasty of hip in connection with osteoarthritis, fractured neck of femur, and 'other diagnoses'"	27,080	Total hip replacement + replacement of head of femur + ?	41,546 + 2,798 + ?	"Other diagnoses" in 1977 category make it broader than data available for recent years.
"Arthroplasty of the hip" including "any replacement or repair operation performed on the hip"	37,290	. . .	. . .	It is not clear which additional procedures (beyond the 27,080) are included here.
"Arthroplasty of hip in connection with fractured neck of femur"	8,630	Replacement of head of femur	2,798	Comparable

Sources: For 1977 data see Department of Health and Social Services, *Orthopaedic Services: Waiting Times for Outpatient Appointments and Inpatient Treatment*. Report of a Working Party to the Secretary of State for Social Services (London: Her Majesty's Stationery Office, 1981). The 2000 data are from Department of Health, Hospital Episode Statistics 2001, table 5 (www.dh.gov.uk/PublicationsAndStatistics/Statistics/HospitalEpisode Statistics/fs/en [June 2005]).

a. "2000" data are for *fiscal year* 2000—the last six months of 1999 and first six months of 2000.

admissions and treatments. Both emergency and nonemergency admissions were likely included in the 1977 statistics. Nevertheless, separate statistics are shown for both groups of patients in table A-3.

Hip replacement operations clearly are more common in Britain today than they were in 1977. How much more common is unclear. If one

Table A-3. *Hip Replacement Procedures Performed in Britain, 1977 and 2000*[a]

Units as indicated

Procedure	1977	1999– 2000 (non- emer- gency)	Percent change	1999– 2000 (all admis- sions)	Percent change
Total hip replacement					
Number performed	14,200	41,546	193	45,841	223
Rate per million	286	845	196	933	226
Rate per million age 60+	1,398	4,073	191	4,495	221
Replacement of head of femur					
Number performed	8,630	2,798	–68	21,826	153
Rate per million	174	57	–67	444	155
Rate per million age 60+	850	274	–68	2,140	152
All hip replacements					
Number performed	22,830	44,344	94	67,667	196
Rate per million	460	902	96	1,377	199
Rate per million age 60+	2,248	4,348	93	6,634	195

Sources: Department of Health, *Orthopaedic Services*, p. 20; *Hospital Episode Statistics 2001*, table 5.

a. "2000" data are for *fiscal year* 2000 (1999–2000). Data for 1977 are for England and Wales, while 1999–2000 figures are for England only.

assumes that the earlier data captured hip operations performed on patients admitted as regular inpatients, as well as on those admitted through emergency departments, the population-adjusted rate of hip operations has increased about 200 percent. But if one assumes that the earlier data excluded patients admitted through emergency departments, the increase is closer to 100 percent. Similarly, the population-adjusted rate of total hip replacement has jumped between 191 and 221 percent over this period, depending on which breakdown of the recent statistics is compared.

The biggest uncertainties involve partial hip replacements. Trends in the frequency of operations involving the "replacement of head of femur" vary markedly depending on which breakdown of the 2000 data is used. Partial operations performed on all patients, regardless of whether they were admitted as emergency or nonemergency cases, increased over 150 percent since 1977. But partial replacement operations on patients who

Table A-4. *Ratio of Hip Operations in Britain versus the United States, Late 1970s and 2000, in the Population Age Sixty and Over*

Procedure	Late 1970s[a]	2000[b]
Option 1: All admissions[c]		
Total hip replacement	0.69	1.04
Partial hip replacement	0.41	0.90
All hip replacements	0.55	0.99
Option 2: Nonemergency[d]		
Total hip replacement	0.69	0.94
Partial hip replacement	0.41	0.11
All hip replacements	0.55	0.65

Sources: Calculated from rate per million age 60+, tables A-1 and A-3.

a. U.S. data are for 1979; British data are for 1977.

b. U.S. figures for 2000 include all operations, whether patients were admitted on an emergency or nonemergency basis.

c. Recent British data under this category include all operations, whether patients were admitted as emergency or nonemergency cases.

d. Recent British data under this category include only operations performed on patients admitted as regular (nonemergency) inpatients.

are admitted as regular, nonemergency cases fell about 68 percent. Such a drop seems anomalous, as demand for partial hip replacements has almost certainly increased since 1977. For that reason it seems likely that the 1977 statistics included both emergency and nonemergency operations. Partial replacement operations are often performed in patients with broken hips or other accidental injuries who are admitted through emergency departments. If the 1977 data included partial replacements, eliminating emergency admissions from the recent data would likely lead to such a seemingly anomalous decline in partial hip operations.

Cross-National Comparisons over Time

Table A-4 shows the ratio of total and partial hip replacement operations in the older population in Britain as compared to the United States, both on an emergency and all-admissions basis, over the past two decades.

Notes

Chapter One

1. Kevin Murphy and Robert Topel, eds., *Measuring the Gains from Medical Research: An Economic Approach* (University of Chicago Press, 2003); David M. Cutler and Mark McClellan, "Is Technological Change in Medicine Worth It?" *Health Affairs* 20, no. 5 (2001): 11–29.

2. Historical data from Centers on Medicare and Medicaid Services, "Historical National Health Expenditures by Type of Service and Source of Funds: Calendar Years 1960–02" (www.cms.hhs.gov/statistics/nhe/#download [June 2005]); Stephen Heffler and others, "U.S. Health Spending Projections for 2004–2014," *Health Affairs*, February 23, 2005 (content.healthaffairs.org/cgi/reprint/hlthaff.w5.74v1.pdf [June 2005]).

3. Henry J. Aaron and Jack Meyer, "Health," in *Restoring Fiscal Sanity, 2005*, edited by Alice M. Rivlin and Isabel Sawhill (Brookings, 2005), pp. 73–97.

4. Data on computer purchases from Bureau of Economic Analysis, "Table 2.4.5. Personal Consumption Expenditures by Type of Product," and "Table 2.4.4. Price Indexes for Personal Consumption Expenditures by Type of Product," *National Income and Product Accounts Tables* (www.bea.dot.gov/bea/dn/nipaweb/index.asp [June 2005]).

5. Centers on Medicare and Medicaid Services, "Table 3: National Health Expenditures, by Source of Funds and Type of Expenditure: Selected Calendar Years 1998–2003," *National Health Expenditures Tables* (www.cms.hhs.gov/statistics/nhe/historical [June 2005]).

6. David Cutler, *Your Money or Your Life: Strong Medicine for America's Health Care System* (Oxford University Press, December 2003); Cutler and McClellan, "Technological Change in Medicine."

7. Victor R. Fuchs and Alan M. Garber, "Health and Medical Care," in *Agenda for the Nation,* edited by Henry J. Aaron, James Lindsay, and Pietro Nivola (Brookings, 2003), pp. 172–73.

8. Ann Meadow, "Access to Care under Physician Payment Reform: A Physician-Based Analysis—Access to Health Services for Vulnerable Populations," *Health Care Financing Review* 17, no. 2 (1995): 195–217; *Senior Journal,* "Brief History of the Medicare Program" (www.seniorjournal.com/NEWS/2000% 20Files/Aug%2000/FTR-08-04-00MedCarHistry.htm [June 2005]).

9. Organization for Economic Cooperation and Development, *OECD Health Data 2004,* 3rd ed. (Paris, June 2004). Following Switzerland as the next highest in per capita spending on health care are Norway ($3,409), Luxembourg ($3,065), and Canada ($2,931).

10. In a review of many studies of the relationship between per capita income and per capita health care spending, Ulf-G. Gerdtham and Bengt Jönsson conclude, "A common and extremely robust result of international comparisons is that the effect of per capita GDP (income) on expenditure is clearly positive and significant and, further, that the estimated income elasticity is clearly higher than zero and close to unity or even higher than unity." See Ulf-G. Gerdtham and Bengt Jönsson, "International Comparisons of Health Expenditure: Theory, Data, and Econometric Analysis," in *Handbook of Health Economics,* vol. 1A, edited by Anthony J. Culyer and Joseph P. Newhouse (New York: Elsevier, 2000), p. 45. That is, health care spending is a constant or rising proportion of income as per capita income rises. For a higher estimate, see Uwe Reinhardt, Peter Hussey, and Gerard Anderson, "U.S. Health Care Spending in an International Context," *Health Affairs* 23, no. 1 (2004): 10–25.

11. Great Britain includes England, Wales, and Scotland; the United Kingdom includes Northern Ireland as well. In this book some data refer to England, some to England and Wales, some to Great Britain (that is, England, Wales, and Scotland), and some to the United Kingdom. "Great Britain" is used as the general term to avoid confusion; where precision of reference is necessary, the correct entity is used in the text or in a footnote.

12. For data on U.S. hospital expenditures, see Centers on Medicare and Medicaid Services, "Table 3"; for data on U.S. population, see Census Bureau, "Time Series of National Population Estimates," July 31, 2002 (www.census.gov/ popest/archives/2000s/vintage_2002/NA-EST2002-01.html [June 2005]). For data on U.K. hospital expenditures, see Department of Health, "Departmental Report 2004" (London, April 2004), p. 88 (www.dh.gov.uk/PublicationsAnd Statistics/Publications/AnnualReports/fs/en [June 2005]); for data on U.K. population, see Office of National Statistics, "Census 2001: Profiles: England" (www. statistics.gov.uk/census2001/profiles/64.asp [June 2005]). Conversion to dollars is based on an exchange rate of £0.69 per U.S. dollar as of January 2, 2002. See Federal Reserve, "Foreign Exchange Rates" (www.federalreserve.gov/releases/ g5a/20020102/ [June 2005]).

13. The menu of services examined in these chapters overlaps but is not identical to that of *The Painful Prescription: Rationing Hospital Care,* published over

two decades ago (Brookings, 1984). Many services have changed or been supplemented. Coronary artery surgery has been joined by percutaneous transluminal angioplasty for treatment of occluded coronary arteries. The field of radiology has been transformed by new equipment. Treatment of cancer has become so varied and sophisticated that brief summaries and comparisons of the highly differentiated care of different tumors have become impossible.

14. See "Dartmouth Atlas of Health Care" (www.dartmouthatlas.org [June 2005]). See also Jonathan Skinner, Elliott Fisher, and John E. Wennberg, "The Efficiency of Medicare," Working Paper 8395 (Cambridge, Mass.: National Bureau of Economic Research, July 2001).

15. Victor Fuchs amusingly ridicules the idea that defensive medicine is not practiced. See Victor Fuchs, "Physician-Induced Demand: A Parable," *Journal of Health Economics* 5, no. 4 (1986): 367.

Chapter Two

1. Organization for Economic Cooperation and Development (OECD), *OECD Health Data 2002*, 4th ed. (Paris, 2002).

2. Ibid. Comparisons of doctors and nurses in the United States and United Kingdom are for 1999, based on purchasing power parities. Comparisons of acute care beds are for 2000.

3. In the year 2000, life expectancy at birth for newborn girls and boys in England and Wales exceeded that in the United states by 0.7 and 1.3 years, respectively. Newborns in 2000 died at the rate of 5.6 per thousand in Great Britain and 6.9 per thousand in the United States. See Office for National Statistics, *Mortality Statistics—General: Review of the Registrar General on Deaths in England and Wales, 2000*, Series DH1 no. 33 (London, 2002), p. 98, and *Mortality Statistics—Childhood, Infant and Perinatal: Review of the Registrar General on Deaths in England and Wales, 2000*, Series DH3, no. 33 (London, 2002), p. 46; Elizabeth Arias, "United States Life Tables, 2000," *National Vital Statistics Reports* 51, no. 3 (December 19, 2002): 29; T. J. Mathews, Fay Menacker, and Marian F. MacDorman, "Infant Mortality Statistics from the 2000 Period Linked Birth/Infant Death Data Set," *National Vital Statistics Reports* 50, no. 12 (August 28, 2002), p. 11.

4. Victor Fuchs and Alan Garber, "Health and Medical Care," in *Agenda for the Nation*, edited by Henry J. Aaron, James M. Lindsay, and Pietro S. Nivola, (Brookings, 2003), pp. 145–81; Victor Fuchs, *Who Shall Live? Health, Economics and Social Choice* (Singapore: World Scientific, 1998).

5. Howard Glennerster, *British Social Policy since 1945* (Oxford: Blackwell, 1995), pp. 3–4, 45–54; Economic Models Limited and American Medical Association, *The British Health Care System* (Chicago, 1976), pp. 31, 35.

6. Geoffrey Rivett, *From Cradle to Grave: Fifty Years of NHS History* (London: King's Fund, 1998); Charles Webster, *The National Health Services since the War*, vol. 1 (London: Stationery Office, 1998), chapter 2; Glennerster, *British Social Policy since 1945*, p. 47.

7. Manfred Huber and Eva Orosz, "Health Expenditure Trends in OECD Countries," *Health Care Financing Review* 25, no. 1 (2003): 1–22; Webster, *National Health Service*, p. 802. Expenditure in the United Kingdom for 1954 excludes out-of-pocket payments; expenditure for 1980 does not.

8. Health expenditure in the U.S. in 1960 is taken from *OECD Health Data 2002*, 4th ed. Data for 2003 are from the Center for Medicare and Medicaid Services, "Table 1: National Health Expenditures Aggregate and per Capita Amounts, Percent Distribution, and Average Annual Percent Growth, by Source of Funds: Selected Calendar Years 1980–2003" (www.cms.hhs.gov/statistics/nhe/historical/t1.asp [June 2005]).

9. In 1960, 11.7 percent of the U.K. population and 9.2 percent of the U.S. population were sixty-five years of age or over. The comparable figures for these two countries in 2000 were 15.8 percent and 12.3 percent, respectively. See *OECD Health Data 2002*, 4th ed.

10. Rivett, *From Cradle to Grave*.

11. In 1949 the NHS handled 2.9 million inpatient cases, and this figure rose to 5.9 million in 1967. Data for 1949 from Rivett, "1948–1957: Establishing the National Health Service," *From Cradle to Grave*. Data on later years from *OECD Health Data 2002*, 4th ed.

12. Henry Aaron and William Schwartz, *The Painful Prescription: Rationing Hospital Care* (Brookings, 1984).

13. Julian Le Grand, Nicholas Mays, and Jo-Ann Mulligan, *Learning from the N.H.S. Internal Market: A Review of the Evidence* (London: King's Fund, 1997). On possible negative consequences of competition without adequate quality indicators, see Carol Propper, Simon Burgess, and Katherine Greene, "Does Competition between Hospitals Improve Quality of Care? Hospital Death Rates and the N.H.S. Internal Market," *Journal of Public Economics* 88, no. 7-8 (2004): 1247–72. These authors found that death rates from acute myocardial infarction increased in competitive areas, even as costs fell. In contrast, Bernard Dowling reports that fundholding competition reduced waiting times; see Bernard Dowling, *GPs and Purchasing in the NHS: The Internal Market and Beyond* (Aldershot and Brookfield, Vt.: Ashgate, 2000). See also Howard Glennerster and others, *Implementing GP Fundholding: Wild Card or Winning Hand* (Philadelphia: Open University Press, 1994).

14. H.M. Treasury, "Delivering High Quality Public Services," *Budget Report 2003* (London: Stationery Office, April 2003), chap. 6, p. 150.

15. The funding increases for the NHS were promised in H.M. Treasury, *Budget Report 2000* (London: Stationery Office, 2000); and H.M. Treasury, *Budget Report 2003*, p. 145.

16. Derek Wanless, *Securing Our Future Health: Taking a Long-Term View, Final Report* (H.M. Treasury, April 2002).

17. Insurance also influences innovation. Since patients bear little of the expense of costly innovations, health care research can be biased toward the development of higher quality and more costly procedures than is socially optimal, rather than lower cost or cost-reducing innovations. Fuchs and Garber, *Agenda for the Nation*.

18. Some of the British seem to identify "equity" with "equality." See, for example, Adam Wagstaff and Eddy van Doorslaer, "Equity in Health Care Finance and Delivery," and Alan Williams and Richard Cookson, "Equity in Health," in *Handbook of Health Economics*, vol. 1B, edited by Anthony J. Culyer and Joseph P. Newhouse (Elsevier, 2000), pp. 1803–62 and 1863–910, respectively.

19. Department of Health, *Departmental Report 2003* (London: Stationery Office, March 2003), p. 37.

20. Anna Dixon and Ray Robinson, "The United Kingdom," in *Health Care Systems in Eight Countries: Trends and Challenges*, edited by Anna Dixon and Elias Mossialos (London: European Observatory on Health Care Systems, April 2002), pp. 103–14.

21. The national government protected fundholders from unusually large losses by retaining responsibility for costs exceeding an annual maximum. Hospitals, which formerly had been under the direct control of local health authorities, became managerially independent, with their own governing bodies. But they remained financially dependent on contracts from GP fundholders and on budgets from district health authorities who were loath to see hospitals go bankrupt. The national government also continued to finance hospitals' capital costs.

22. Department of Health, *Statistics for General Medical Practitioners in England 1994–2004*, Statistical Bulletin 2005/02 (London: Stationery Office, 2005), tables 1b and 3.

23. Ibid., p. 10.

24. In June 2004, 83,054 patients' names had been on the English outpatient waiting list for thirteen or more weeks, 3,390 for seventeen or more weeks, and 2,962 for twenty-one or more weeks. Department of Health, "Waiting Times for 1st Outpatient Appointments, Quarter 1 2004/2005" (www.performance.doh.gov.uk/waitingtimes/2004/q1/qm08_y00.html [June 2005]).

25. John Appleby and Anna Coote, eds., *Five-Year Health Check: A Review of Government Health Policy 1997–2002* (London: King's Fund, 2002), p. 21.

26. Contemporary statistics in this section are drawn from King's Fund, *An Independent Audit of the NHS under Labour, 1997–2005*, briefing paper (London, March 2005).

27. Other delays occur between onset of illness and actual treatment: delays in seeing GPs, delays between being seen by a GP and being placed on the outpatient list, delays between being seen as an outpatient and being placed on the inpatient list, and delays in treatment after admission.

28. A survey of the National Audit Office revealed that nearly half of the hospital chief executives responding had redefined how they counted inpatients in 1999–2000, following the announcement of new waiting list targets. This would include, for example, reclassifying patients on the waiting list as "planned" admissions, which are not counted on the inpatient waiting list. Nearly all reported reclassifications of patients led to a reduction in the number of people on inpatient waiting lists. National Audit Office, *Inpatient and Outpatient Waiting in the HS* (London: Stationery Office, 2001), p. 20.

29. Department of Health, "Cancer Waiting Times: England Summary" (www.performance.doh.gov.uk/cancerwaits/2004/q4/eng.html [June 2005]).

30. Stephen Frankel and Robert West, eds., *Rationing and Rationality in the National Health Service: The Persistence of Waiting Lists* (London: Macmillan, 1993), p. 22; National Audit Office, *Inpatient and Outpatient Waiting,* p. 2.

31. King's Fund, *Independent Audit,* p. 29

32. Department of Health and Social Security, *Priorities in Health and Social Services* (London: HMSO, 1977), p.7.

33. Howard Glennerster and others. *Paying for Health, Education, and Housing: How Does the Centre Pull the Purse Strings?* (Oxford University Press, 2000), p. 73.

34. Carol Propper and Richard Upward, "Need, Equity and the NHS: The Distribution of Health Care Expenditure 1974–1987," *Fiscal Studies* 13, no. 2, (1992): 1–21.

35. Department of Health, *Independent Inquiry into Inequalities in Health: The Acheson Report* (London: Stationery Office, 1998).

36. Audit Commission, *A Focus on General Practice in England* (London, 2002), p. 49.

37. For data on the number of pay beds in the NHS, see House of Commons Health Committee, *First Report Session 2001–2002* (Stationery Office, May 2001); for the total number of acute beds in the United Kingdom, see *OECD Health Data 2002,* 4th ed.; and for the number of acute beds in the independent sector, see Laing and Buisson, *Laing's Healthcare Market Review 2000–2001* (London, 2001), p. 62. The number of acute inpatient beds in the NHS is calculated as the number of acute beds in the United Kingdom minus the number of acute beds in the independent sector.

38. For the number of private hospitals and the number of beds in private hospitals, see Laing and Buisson, *Healthcare Market Review,* p. 62; for the number of NHS pay beds, see House of Commons Health Committee, *First Report.* The total number of acute inpatient beds available for private care is taken as the sum of NHS beds and beds in private hospitals. This is a high-end estimate because a small minority of beds in private hospitals are used by the NHS, primarily for psychiatric care, care of the elderly, and abortions. Less than 1 percent of patients having elective surgery in the private sector had their operation financed by public funds. Yvonne Doyle and Adrian Bull, "Role of Private Sector in the United Kingdom Healthcare System," *British Medical Journal* 321 (September 2, 2002), p. 563–65.

39. Brian Williams and others, "Private Funding of Elective Hospital Treatment in England and Wales, 1997–8: National Survey," *British Medical Journal* 320 (April 1, 2000): 904–05; Elias Mossialos and Sarah Thomson, "Voluntary Health Insurance in the European Union: A Critical Assessment," *International Journal of Health Services* 32, no. 1 (2002): 19–88.

40. Doyle and Bull, "Role of the Private Sector," p. 563.

41. These values are for 1999. For data on private expenditure, see Laing and Buisson, *Healthcare Market Review,* p. 52; for spending on inpatient and outpatient care and physicians, referred to as "hospital, community health and family health services" expenditure, see Department of Health, *The Government's Expenditure Plans 2000–2001: Departmental Report 2000* (London: Stationery

Office, 2000), Annex B; and for total health expenditure, see *OECD Health Data 2002*, 4th ed. The OECD source reports that private outlays constituted 19 percent of total health spending in 2000, but this figure appears to include nonprescription pharmacy purchases.

42. Of eighty-six units with 1,414 beds within the NHS dedicated to private patients, twenty-five units with 609 beds were within Greater London. Laing and Buisson, *Healthcare Market Review*, p. 68. Only one Scot in twenty-five had private insurance coverage.

43. In 1996, 22 percent of professionals and 23 percent of employers and managers had private coverage. Derek King and Elias Mossialos, *The Determinants of Private Medical Insurance Prevalence in England*, Health and Social Care Discussion Paper 3 (London School of Economics, May 2002), p. 1; Elias Mossialos and Sarah M. S. Thomson, "Voluntary Health Insurance in the European Union: A Critical Assessment," *International Journal of Health Services*, 32, no. 1 (2002): 19–88.

44. Rose Wiles and Joan Higgins, *Why Do Patients Go Private? A Study of Consumerism in Healthcare* (Southampton: Institute for Policy Studies, 1992). The authors point out that actual waits were much shorter than patients believed them to be.

45. Office of Fair Trading, *Health Insurance* (London, July 1996).

46. Laing and Buisson, *Healthcare Market Review*, p. 89.

47. CareHealth, "Private Medical Insurance Explained" (www.carehealth.co.uk/pmiexpln.htm#addons [June 2005]).

48. One reason for the rapid growth of private insurance premiums was the 1989 Health and Medicines Act, which authorized NHS hospitals to charge private patients market prices. Between 1988 and 1992, NHS income from private patient units increased by 40 percent. Competition Commission, "Private Medical Services: A Report on Agreements and Practices Relating to Charges for the Supply of Private Medical Services by NHS Consultants" (London, 1994). See also Rivett, *From Cradle to Grave*.

49. One policy offered by BUPA, the United Kingdom's largest private insurer, offered 3,960 variants of a single policy and 114 different monthly premium options. Office of Fair Trading, *Health Insurance*; "Final Warning to Health Insurers," press release, May 28,1998 (www.oft.gov.uk/News/Press+releases/1998/PN+27-98.htm [June 2005]); and "Health Insurance: A Second Report from the Office of Fair Trading" (London, May 1998). See also CareHealth, "Criticisms of Private Medical Insurance by the Office of Fair Trading" (www.carehealth.co.uk/pmicrit.htm [June 2005]).

50. Laing and Buisson, *Healthcare Market Review*, p. 140–41.

51. This practice was described by foreign physicians who have practiced in Great Britain and was acknowledged by British general practitioners.

52. An anonymous reviewer of this manuscript wrote, "I am not aware of U.S. physicians who will refuse to do an angioplasty along with a cardiac catheterization because of reimbursement benefits. I have, however, seen gastroenterologists refuse to do an upper and a lower GI [gastrointestinal] endoscopy study to increase the amount they can bill by doing them separately."

53. Individual coverage for a 50-year-old man is available from U.K. insurer AXA PPP starting at $48 per month, while the least expensive plan for a 50-year-old in the United States is around $170. For U.K. rates, see CareHealth, "Criticisms of Private Medical Insurance." U.S. rate quotes are from www.ehealthin-surance.com [June 2005]. Monetary conversion is based on an exchange rate of $1 = £0.54, as of November 15, 2004 (www.federalreserve.gov/releases/h10/20041115 [June 2005]).

54. The average pay for American doctors was 5.5 times the average wage in the 1996 OECD cross-country data, whereas doctors in the United Kingdom make only 1.4 times the average wage. See Uwe E. Reinhardt, Peter S. Hussey, and Gerard F. Anderson, "Cross-National Comparisons of Health Systems Using OECD Data, 1999," *Health Affairs* 21, no. 3 (2002): 169–81. See also Mossialos and Thomson, "Voluntary Health Insurance."

55. The low occupancy rates resulted partly from the superior amenities available for minor procedures in privately owned facilities and from the hostility of some NHS hospital employees toward private patients, as well as from shortened average stays and increased charges. See Royal Commission on the National Health Service, *Report of the Royal Commission* (London: HMSO, 1979), p. 291; Michael Lee, *Private and National Health Services* (London: Policy Studies Institute, 1978), p. 12.

56. Clifford Krauss, "In Blow to Canada's Health System, Quebec Law Is Voided," *New York Times*, June 10, 2005.

57. Ninety percent of all contacts with the NHS get no further than the GP. Howard Glennerster, *Understanding the Finance of Welfare* (Bristol: Policy Press, 2003), p. 56.

Chapter Three

1. G. Pincherle, *Topics of Our Time, 2: Kidney Transplants and Dialysis* (London: Her Majesty's Stationery Office, 1979), p. 25.

2. Personal communication from Dr. Marcos Rothstein, Washington University School of Medicine, St. Louis, 2004.

3. Data from U.S. Renal Data System, *USRDS 2003 Annual Data Report: Atlas of End-Stage Renal Disease in the United States* (Bethesda, Md.: National Institutes of Health [NIH], National Institute of Diabetes and Digestive and Kidney Diseases [NIDDK], 2003). These annual data reports can be accessed at www.usrds.org.

4. U.S. Renal Data System, *USRDS 2004 Annual Data Report: Atlas of End-Stage Renal Disease in the United States* (Bethesda, Md.: NIH, NIDDK, 2004).

5. David Ansell and Terry Feest, eds., *U.K. Renal Registry Report 2001* (Bristol, U.K.: U.K. Renal Registry, December 2001), chap. 9.

6. Philip F. Halloran, "Immunosuppressive Drugs for Kidney Transplantation," *New England Journal of Medicine* 351, no. 26 (2004): 2715–29. The first immunosuppressive agent, azathioprine, was first used in clinical trials in 1962 but was displaced by cyclosporin. See also National Research Development Corporation, "Cyclosporin 'A'" (www.nrdcindia.com/pages/sporin.htm [June 2005]).

7. For first-year failure rates, see H. Krakauer and others, "The Recent U.S. Experience in the Treatment of End-Stage Renal Disease by Dialysis and Transplantation," *New England Journal of Medicine* 308, no. 26 (1983): 1558–63. The failure rates after one year, five years, and ten years are 6, 21, and 45 percent, respectively, for transplants from living donors. The corresponding failure rates for cadaveric transplants are 11, 34, and 64 percent, respectively. Mohamed H. Sayegh and Charles B. Carpenter, "Transplantation 50 Years Later—Progress, Challenges, and Promises," *New England Journal of Medicine* 351, no. 26 (2004): 2761–66, table 1.

8. Halloran, "Immunosuppressive Drugs for Kidney Transplantation." Research now indicates that some immunosuppressive drugs predispose patients to the development of various cancers; switching to other drugs reverses this process. Giovanni Stallone and others, "Sirolimus for Kaposi's Sarcoma in Renal-Transplant Recipients," *New England Journal of Medicine* 352, no. 13 (2005): 1317–23; Jacques Dantal and Jean-Paul Soulillou, "Immunosuppressive Drugs and the Risk of Cancer after Organ Transplantation," *New England Journal of Medicine* 352, no. 13 (2005): 1371–73.

9. Sayegh and Carpenter, "Transplantation 50 Years Later." Mortality rates may be higher in the United States than in Europe in part because patients accepted for treatment in the United States are older and sicker than is typical elsewhere. There are also some indications that adverse events may be underreported in Europe. Stephen Pastan and James Bailey, "Dialysis Therapy," *New England Journal of Medicine* 338, no. 20 (1998): 1428–36.

10. Organization for Economic Cooperation and Development (OECD), *OECD Health Data 2002*, 4th ed. (Paris, 2004).

11. One-year mortality rates in Canada were 1 percent each for cadaver and living donor transplants. Graft failure and patient mortality in the United Kingdom are also considerably higher than they are in Australia. Data were analyzed by the U.K. Transplant Authority and provided by personal communication from David Ansell, director, U.K. Renal Registry, Bristol, November 10, 2003.

12. Sayegh and Carpenter, "Transplantation 50 Years Later."

13. The number of deaths for waiting list patients in Britain is from NHS, U.K. Transplant, *More Transplants—New Lives: Transplant Activity U.K. 2003–2004* (Bristol, U.K., September 2004), p. 13. Data on the number of deaths for waiting list patients in the United States are from the Organ Procurement and Transplantation Network, "National Data Reports" (www.optn.org [July 2005]). The number of donors has declined in the United Kingdom over the past decade. As a result the number of names on the waiting list has increased about 3 percent annually since 1994. In March 2003 there were over 5,000 names on the waiting list for kidney transplants in the United Kingdom. See U.K. Transplant, *More Transplants,* p. 13.

14. Medicare Payment Advisory Commission, *Report to the Congress: New Approaches in Medicare* (Washington, June 2004), p. 58.

15. In 1979 hospital, center, and home hemodialysis cost $52,524, $42,019, and $31,514, respectively, when adjusted for inflation. Eighty-seven percent of dialysis was done in hospitals or centers. See H. Krakauer and others, "Recent

U.S. Experience"; Asad A. Bakir and George Dunea, "Current Trends in the Treatment of Uraemia: A View from the United States," *British Medical Journal* 1 (April 7, 1979): 914–16; Office of Health Economics, *Renal Failure: A Priority in Health?* (London, 1978), pp. 42–43; Pincherle, *Topics of Our Time*, p. 16; and Gordon Scorer and Anthony Wing, eds., *Decision Making in Medicine: The Practice of Its Ethics* (London: Edward Arnold, 1979), p. 161.

16. Cost of dialysis in the U.K. is from Graham Mowatt and others, *Systematic Review of the Effectiveness and Cost-Effectiveness of Home versus Hospital or Satellite Unit Haemodialysis for People with End-Stage Renal Failure* (Aberdeen, Scotland: Health Services Research Unit, University of Aberdeen, April 2, 2002), p. 94. These costs for hemodialysis assume three sessions per week. The estimates include access (insertion) costs, equipment and building costs (including estimates of the cost of necessary home conversion for home hemodialysis patients), nursing and medical staff, costs of foreseeable medical complications, and the training costs associated with home hemodialysis. Note: currency conversion is based on a 2001 exchange rate of $1.44 per British pound.

17. The higher U.S. estimate of $115,000 comes from Roger W. Evans and Daniel J. Kitzman, "An Economic Analysis of Kidney Transplantation," *Surgical Clinics of North America* 78, no. 1 (1998): 149–74. The lower figure of $95,000 is an estimate for 2001 taken from the U.S. Renal Data System, *USRDS 2002 Annual Data Report: Atlas of End-Stage Renal Disease in the United States* (Bethesda, Md.: NIH, NIDDK, 2002), p. 27. The cost of kidney transplants in Britain is for the fiscal year 2001–02. See Department of Health, *NHS Reference Costs 2002* (London, 2003), appendix 1A, procedure L01. Procedural cost of a kidney transplant includes staff and equipment but does not include hospital costs, which vary with a patient's length of stay.

18. British physicians also speculate that financial incentives in the United States, together with physicians' fears of being sued, may cause excessive dialysis of patients whose quality of life is poor and who in Britain would be provided pain relief or sedation and be allowed to die.

19. One consultant nephrologist candidly acknowledged, "I must create propaganda in my unit which puts pressure on patients not to get stuck on the limited hospital dialysis facilities but to submit themselves and their families to the incessant demands of home dialysis or volunteer for transplantation." Scorer and Wing, eds., *Decision Making in Medicine*, p. 161.

20. For more information on treatment of kidney failure around 1980, see Henry J. Aaron and William B. Schwartz, *The Painful Prescription* (Brookings, 1984).

21. For British data see David Ansell and others, eds., *U.K. Renal Registry Report 2003* (Bristol, U.K.: U.K. Renal Registry, December 2003). U.S. data are from U.S. Renal Data System, *2004 Annual Data Report*, table D-1.

22. Ansell and others, *Renal Registry Report 2003*; U.S. Renal Data System, *2004 Annual Data Report*, table D-4.

23. P. J. Boyle, H. Kudlac, and A. J. Williams, "Geographic Variation in the Referral of Patients with Chronic End Stage Renal Failure for Renal Replacement Therapy," *Quarterly Journal of Medicine* 89, no. 2 (1996): 151–57. An older

study had reached similar conclusions. See Maureen Dalziel and Chris Garrett, "Intraregional Variation in Treatment of End Stage Renal Failure," *British Medical Journal* 294 (May 30, 1987): 1382–83.

24. British Kidney Alliance, *End Stage Renal Failure: A Framework for Planning and Service Delivery: Towards Equity and Excellence in Renal Services* (London, January 2001), p. 24.

25. Ibid., p. 39.

26. Increases in acceptance rates for patients over age sixty-five were noted in David Ansell and Terry Feest, eds., *U.K. Renal Registry Report 1999* (Bristol, U.K.: U.K. Renal Registry, December 1999), p. 3.

27. In 2000, 6.3 percent of the U.S. population were diabetic. The comparable percentage for England is 2.6. See Sarah Wild and others, "Global Prevalence of Diabetes: Estimates for the Year 2000 and Projections for 2030," *Diabetes Care* 27, no. 5 (2004): 1047–53; Department of Health, *National Service Framework for Diabetes: One Year On* (London, 2004), p. 1.

28. According to the U.S. Renal Data System online database, 45.6 percent of patients accepted for dialysis in 2000 were diabetic. U.S. Renal Data System, *USRDS 2000 Annual Data Report: Atlas of End-Stage Renal Disease in the United States* (Bethesda, Md.: NIH, NIDDK, 2000). The U.K. Renal Registry reports that in 2002, 18 percent of newly accepted patients for dialysis were diabetic. See David Ansell and others, *Renal Registry Report 2003* . According to one British nephrologist, 60 percent of Asians (Pakistanis and Indians, in the British context) over age sixty-five in and around Leicester have diabetes.

29. Personal communication from Dr. Marcos Rothstein. Population data are from Bureau of the Census, "Annual Estimates of the Population by Race Alone and Hispanic or Latino Origin for the United States and States: July 1, 2003" (www.census.gov/popest/states/asrh/tables/SC-EST2003-04.pdf [June 2005]).

30. R. Davies and P. Roderick, "Predicting the Future Demand for RRT in England Using Simulation Modeling," *Nephrology, Dialysis, Transplantation* 12, no. 25 (1997): 2512–16.

31. In 2000 the renal replacement incidence rates per million population—dialysis plus functioning transplants—were 89 in Norway, 93 in the Netherlands, and 94 in Finland, but they were 143 in Canada, 157 in Greece, 175 in Germany, 252 in Japan, and 337 in the United States. British renal replacement rates were comparatively lower, an estimated 91 per million population. U.S. Renal Data System, *Annual Data Report 2002*, figure 13.c, p. 209; David Ansell, Terry Feest, and Catherine Byrne, eds, *U.K. Renal Registry Report 2002* (Bristol. U.K.: U.K. Renal Registry, December 2002), table 4.28, p. 43. One nephrologist expressed full-blown conflict on the issue of age-based rationing: "And if, indeed, we have got lower take-on rates in the 70s and 80s than other continental countries, you know, one has to accept that might be because they never get to see us. It might be that, in fact, my concept of co-morbidity and quality of life is different to those of others, you know, because there is a subjective element to that. And it might be that older U.K. people, if they are told they can't have dialysis, are more likely to accept it than in other countries. . . . But if you spoke to our younger generation of nephrologists, guys under the age of 50, running dialysis programs, they would

be horrified at any suggestion that there was any ageism going on here now. They really would."

32. Tabulations based on data provided by a personal communication from David Ansell, director, U.K. Renal Registry, Bristol, November 4, 2003, and from the U.S. Renal Data System, *2000 Annual Data Report*.

33. In 1996, 41.5 percent of all dialysis patients in the United Kingdom received home dialysis, compared with 15.2 percent in the United States, in part, perhaps, because local authorities relieve the NHS of some minor costs of home dialysis by paying for home assistance—a means-tested disability benefit. OECD, *Health Data 2002*.

34. A foreign physician familiar with the NHS reported that 77 percent of British patients had to wait more than four weeks for the operation to establish a fistula, compared with 5 percent in the United States, 6 percent in Belgium, and zero percent in France.

35. In the words of one nephrologist, "There are a number of relatively simple things I think that could be done. . . . If the serum creatinine was measured in a way that allowed an estimate of the GFR [glomerular filtration rate, a standard measure of kidney function] to be made . . . that would be a major plus for identifying patients at risk of developing renal failure." He also regretted the failure to follow "best practice guidelines for management of hypertension, management of diabetes, and the much more widespread use of ACE [angiotensin-converting enzyme] inhibitors and receptor-blocking drugs."

36. Medicare Payment Advisory Commission, *New Approaches in Medicare*, pp. 58–64.

37. Aaron and Schwartz, *Painful Prescription*, p. 37.

38. For studies of rejection criteria (particularly age), see Frank Kee and others, "Stewardship or Clinical Freedom? Variations in Dialysis Decision Making," *Nephrology, Dialysis, Transplantation* 15, no. 10 (2000): 1647–57. R. G. Parry, A. Crowe, M. Stevens and others, "Referral of Elderly Patients with Severe Renal Failure: Questionnaire Survey of Physicians," *British Medical Journal* 313 (August 24, 1996): 466; A. J. Williams and A. J. Antao, "Referral of Elderly Patients with End-Stage Renal Failure for Renal Replacement Therapy," *Quarterly Journal of Medicine* 72 (August 1989): 749–56; I. H. Khan and others, "Acute Renal Failure: Factors Influencing Nephrology Referral and Outcome," *Quarterly Journal of Medicine* 90 (December 1997): 781–85; Sahid M. Chandna and others, "Is There a Rationale for Rationing Chronic Dialysis? A Hospital-Based Cohort Study of Factors Affecting Survival and Morbidity," *British Medical Journal* 318 (January 23, 1999): 217–23.

39. Medical Services Study Group of the Royal College of Physicians, "Deaths from Chronic Renal Failure under the Age of 50,"*British Medical Journal* 283 (July 25, 1981): 283–86. This conclusion drew heavy fire. A subsequent editorial noted the strong correlation between availability of facilities and numbers of patients treated, suggesting that the distribution of facilities does not match the distribution of renal failure. The editorialist also pointed out the flaw in considering only patients under fifty, because only this cohort receives treatment in near

adequate numbers. See "Audit in Renal Failure," *British Medical Journal* 283 (September 12, 1981): 726–27.

40. Office of Health Economics, *End Stage Renal Failure* (London: White Crescent Press, 1980), pp. 1–8.

41. The proportion of patients accepted for renal replacement therapy who are age sixty-five or older has grown from 11 percent to 41 percent between 1982 and 1995, and the age-specific acceptance rate per million rose from close to zero in 1980 to nearly 300 in 2001, the highest of any age group. Ansell, Feest, and Byrne, *Renal Registry Report 2002*, p. 23. Nonetheless, underprovision is still reported to be greatest among elders. See NHS Health Care Strategy Unit, *A Review of Renal Services* (London, November 1994); E. C. Mulkerrin, "Rationing Renal Replacement Therapy to Older Patients: Agreed Guidelines Are Needed," *Quarterly Journal of Medicine* 93, no. 4 (2000): 253–55.

42. "Audit in Renal Failure."

43. Asked to order factors used in deciding whether a patient might be denied treatment, U.S. and U.K. physicians had almost identical rankings, placing quality of life, mental status, and life expectancy at the top, and age and ability to pay at the bottom in terms of importance. John K. McKenzie and others, "Dialysis Decision Making in Canada, the United States, and the United Kingdom," *American Journal of Kidney Diseases* 31, no. 1 (1998): 12–18.

44. New treatment rates for the elderly varied by a ratio of more than 3 to 1 among health authority regions. Ansell, Feest, and Byrne, *Renal Registry Report 2002*, p. 25. The proportions of elderly patients beginning dialysis who received hemodialysis ranged from a high of 96 percent (versus 4 percent on peritoneal dialysis) in Sunderland to a low of 29 percent on hemodialysis (versus 71 percent on peritoneal dialysis) in Reading. Ibid., p. 325. At day ninety, differences were narrower but still enormous, ranging from under 20 percent on hemodialysis in Cambridge to nearly 80 percent in Hertfordshire, the health authority with the highest proportion of black and Asian patients among regions reporting in 2002. Ibid., p. 326.

45. Nicholas Brook and others, "Renal Transplantation Surgery," *British Medical Journal* 324 (April 6, 2002): S105a.

46. Celia Wight and Bernard, "Shortage of Organs for Transplantation," *British Medical Journal* 312 (April 20, 1996): 989–90.

47. U.S. waiting lists grew from 16,094 in 1993 to 23,494 in 2002. See Organ Procurement and Transplantation Network and the Scientific Registry of Transplant Recipients, *2003 OPTN/SRTR Annual Report: Transplant Data 1993-2002* (www.ustransplant.org/annual_reports/2003/501_ki.pdf [July 2005]). For data on the decline in transplant rates in the United States, see U.S. Renal Data System, *2002 Annual Data Report*, p. 137.

48. Personal communication from Dr. Marcos Rothstein, Washington University Medical School and Barnes-Jewish Dialysis Center, St. Louis, July 7, 2004.

49. Severe hemophiliacs have less than 1 percent of the normal amount of the deficient factor. Moderate hemophiliacs have 1 to 5 percent of the deficient factor. Mild hemophiliacs have more than 5 percent of the deficient factor. See

"Hemophilia" (www.medceu.com/tests/hemophilia.htm [June 2005]). For older sources, see Department of Health, Education, and Welfare, National Institutes of Health, *Study to Evaluate the Supply-Demand Relationship of AHF and PTC through 1980* (HEW, 1977), pp. 6, 16, 21.

50. Pier M. Mannucci and Edward G. D. Tuddenham, "The Hemophilias—From Royal Genes to Gene Therapy," *New England Journal of Medicine* 344, no. 23 (2001): 1773–79.

51. Hemophilia Health Services, "Basic Hemophilia Statistics" (www.accredo health.net/hhs/bleeding_disorders/hemophilia_stats.html [June 2005]).

52. Ibid.

53. Mannucci and Tuddenham, "The Hemophilias."

54. Hemophilia Health Services, "Basic Hemophilia Statistics."

55. Fear that these methods might not entirely forestall infection caused the British to destroy their plasma pool in 1998 and to import blood products from the United States. The British also provided compensation to HIV-infected hemophiliacs. At the urging of patient advocacy groups, the British government provided £10 million in 1987 to establish the Macfarlane Trust, a London-based charitable organization devoted exclusively to providing financial assistance to hemophiliacs who were infected with HIV through NHS-provided blood infusions. A further £25 million was made available to the trust during the 1990s. See Stephen D. Kletter and Peter J. Rankin, "Cost Trends in the Treatment for Hemophilia: Another View," *Thrombosis and Haemostasis* 88 (October 2002): 542–44, citing *The Wall Street Journal*, November 25, 1998, p. A-1; Haemophilia Society, *An Introduction to Haemophilia and Related Bleeding Disorders* (London, 2001), p. 22.

56. The vast majority of clinicians believe that these recombinant factors are safer than plasma-derived products, although there are some skeptics. See, for example, "Hemophilia," *New England Journal of Medicine* 345, no. 14 (2001): 1066–67. There are currently no licensed gene transfer strategies for treating hemophilia, but prospects for their development are excellent. For a summary of gene transfer strategies currently being investigated, see Katherine A. High, "Gene Transfer as an Approach to Treating Hemophilia," *Seminars in Thrombosis and Hemostasis* 29, no. 1 (2003): 107–19. Such liver damage is treated as a result of past practices. "Liver damage, as a result of factor/blood product use in the past several decades, is common in adult hemophiliacs and older teens." Hemophilia of the Sunshine State, "You and Hemophilia" (www.hemophilia.com/consumers/you/index.htm [June 2005]). "More than 50 percent of patients with severe hemophilia who have used the older products have elevations in liver function enzymes." Dimitrios Agaliotis, "Hemophilia, Overview" (www.emedicine.com/med/topic3528.htm [June 23, 2004]).

57. Mannucci and Tuddenham, "The Hemophilias."

58. The World Health Organization has published guidelines for the amount of factor VIII or IX that should be used, depending on the location of the hemorrhage. World Health Organization, *Delivery of Treatment for Haemophilia* (Geneva, 2002), p. 5.

59. Ibid., pp. 4–5 (authors' calculations, based on data from this source).

60. With purified plasma products, hepatic abnormalities may no longer be related to dose. Personal communication. George Broze, hematologist, Washington University, St. Louis, 2004.

61. "Hemophilia."

62. Paul L. F. Giangrande, "Inhibitory Antibodies in Hemophilia," UKHCDO Guidelines (www.medicine.ox.ac.uk/ohc/Inhibi.htm [June 2005]).

63. Note that this method has a serious flaw: it rests on the very strong and dubious assumption that the prevalence and average severity of hemophilia are the same across nations. However, the prevalence and severity of hemophilia both depend on past treatment intensity. If treatment is suboptimal, hemophiliacs will die young, and severe hemophiliacs will die disproportionately. Thus suboptimal treatment will reduce both the number of surviving hemophiliacs and the severity of the extant disease. Countering this effect would be the fact that suboptimal treatment would increase the accumulated trauma of surviving patients and the likely frequency and severity of bleeds. The strength of these effects is impossible to assess.

64. Both nations far exceed the standard for optimal survival of at least 1 unit per person. However, usage in both nations falls far below that in Germany—5.5 units—as it did two decades ago. Data for the United States are taken from Paula H. B. Bolton-Maggs and K. John Pasi, "Haemophilias A and B," *Lancet* 361 (May 24, 2003): 1801–09. Data for the United Kingdom were provided in a personal communication from Mark Brooker, World Federation of Hemophilia, Montreal, Canada, 2004.

Average use of treatment factors per patient in New York in 1998 was greater than that reported for the entire United Kingdom in 2001. Per patient use of missing factors averaged 89,494 units in New York during 1998 and 64,733 units in the United Kingdom in 2001. However, average use in New York varied from 839,709 units for severe hemophiliacs on prophylaxis with inhibitor immune tolerance to 3,576 units for mild hemophiliacs not on prophylaxis without inhibitors. See Jeanne V. Linden and others, "Factor Concentrate Usage in Persons with Hemophilia in New York State," *Transfusion* 43 (April 2003): 470–75; United Kingdom Haemophilia Centre Doctors' Organisation, *National Haemophilia Database: Report on the Annual Returns for 2000 and 2001* (Manchester, U.K., 2003).

65. Hemophilia Health Services, "Basic Hemophilia Statistics." In 2000 Medicare paid $0.46 to $1.37 per unit for factor VIII and from $0.46 to $0.91 per unit of factor IX. At the lowest price per unit, the average cost of episodic treatment for all patients requiring factor VIII would range from $12,880 to $48,300 a year. The cost of prophylactic treatment would range from $52,232 to $196,320 a year. Medicare price information from Centers for Medicare and Medicaid Services, "Proposed CY 2004: Hospital Outpatient Prospective Payment System," www.cms.hhs.gov/regulations/hopps/2004p/changecy2004.asp? (August 2005).

66. Jeremy Wight and Mike Richards, "Very High Cost Treatment for a Single Individual—A Case Report," *Journal of Public Health Medicine* 25, no.1 (2003): 4–7; Giangrande, "Inhibitory Antibodies."

67. Such an increase could be foreseen. See Aaron and Schwartz, *Painful Prescription*, p. 40. For recent data, see Centers for Disease Control, *Report on the Universal Data Collection Program* 4, no. 2 (2002): 12. An additional survey of American hemophilia treatment centers undertaken in 2000 turned up similar results, finding that one-third of severe hemophiliacs in the United States received long-term prophylaxis. Regina Butler, Wilma McClure, and Karen Wulff, "Practice Patterns in Haemophilia A Therapy—A Survey of Treatment Centres in the United States," *Haemophilia* 9, no. 5 (2003): 549–54.

68. Alexander H. Miners and others, "Financing the Rising Cost of Haemophilia Care at a Large Comprehensive Care Centre," *Journal of the Royal College of Physicians of London* 31, no. 6 (1997): 640–44. See also Haemophilia Society, *Introduction to Haemophilia*; Drew Provan and Denise F. O'Shaughnessy, "Recent Advances in Haematology," *British Medical Journal* 318 (April 10, 1999): 991–94.

69. U.S. cost estimates were developed from prevalence statistics and treatment cost figures from Hemophilia Health Services, "Basic Hemophilia Statistics." United Kingdom estimates were based on prevalence and epidemiology data from Haemophilia Centre Doctors' Organisation, *National Haemophilia Database*, tables 4 and 6 for 2001; data on factor usage from the same source, table 8 for 2001; data on costs of factor products from World Federation of Hemophilia (WFH) letter to WHO Expert Committee on the Selection and Use of Essential Medicines (www.wfh.org/Content_Documents/Blood_Safety/Essential_Meds_List_Subm.pdf [June 2005]), and from WFH, *Report on the WFH Global Survey 2002 for National Member Organizations* (Montreal, 2003); and data for dosage estimates were drawn from WFH, *Key Issues in Hemophilia Treatment: Part 1—Products*" (Montreal, April 1998).

70. National Marrow Donor Program, "History of Stem Cell Transplants" (www.marrow.org/NMDP/history_stem_cell_transplants.html [June 2005]).

71. Aplastic Anemia and MDS International Foundation, "The Diseases" (www.aplastic.org/diseases.shtml [June 2005]).

72. *Health A to Z*, "Aplastic Anemia" (www.healthatoz.com [June 2005]).

73. Patients with leukemia were always subjected to total body irradiation in an attempt to eradicate all tumor cells and prevent later recurrence of the disease. Graft rejection occurred rarely in leukemia patients but did occur in about a quarter of patients with aplastic anemia, and in these patients transplantation was usually repeated. Mortimer M. Bortin, Robert Peter Gale, and A. A. Rimm, "Allogeneic Bone Marrow Transplantation for 144 Patients with Severe Aplastic Anemia," *Journal of the American Medical Association* 245, no. 11 (1981): 1132–39.

74. E. Donnall Thomas, "The Role of Marrow Transplantation in the Eradication of Malignant Disease," *Cancer* 49 (May 15, 1982): 1963–69; Robert Peter Gale, "Progress in Bone Marrow Transplantation in Man," *Survey of Immunologic Research* 1, no. 1 (1982): 40–66.

75. See Robert A. Good and Tazim Verjee, "Historical and Current Perspectives on Bone Marrow Transplantation for Prevention and Treatment of Immunodeficiences and Autoimmunities," *Biology of Blood and Marrow Transplantation* 7, no. 3 (2001): 123–35; Peter W. M. Johnson and Kim Orchard, "Bone

Marrow Transplants—New Indications Exploit the Immune Effects of the Transplanted Cells," *British Medical Journal* 235 (August 17, 2002): 348–49; Michael Potter, Carol Black, and Abi Berger, "Bone Marrow Transplantation for Autoimmune Diseases—An Interesting Approach for Patients with Few Alternatives," *British Medical Journal* 318 (March 20, 1999): 750–51.

76. According to the International Bone Marrow Transplant Registry, peripheral blood cells are used in over 95 percent of autologous transplants in adults and 85 percent of transplants for children. Fausto Loberiza Jr., "Report on State of the Art in Blood and Marrow Transplantation," *IBMTR/ABMTR Newsletter* 10, no. 1 (2003): 7–10.

77. Clinicians also discovered that providing a patient with certain bone marrow growth factors could increase the number of stem cells circulating in the bloodstream to a level that, once harvested, would be sufficient for transplantation. T. L. Holyoake and I. M. Franklin, "Bone Marrow Transplants from Peripheral Blood," *British Medical Journal* 309 (July 2, 1994): 4–5; Richard L. Soutar and Derek J. King, "Fortnightly Review: Bone Marrow Transplantation," *British Medical Journal* 310 (January 7, 1995): 31–36; Andrew Duncombe, "ABC of Clinical Haematology: Bone Marrow and Stem Cell Transplantation," *British Medical Journal* 314 (April 19, 1997): 1179.

78. Patients with multiple myeloma and non-Hodgkin's lymphoma received over half of all SCTs performed in North America in 2002, and virtually all of these patients served as their own stem cell donor. A similar pattern emerges for the United Kingdom. See British Society of Blood and Marrow Transplantation, "U.K. Transplant Activity" (www.bsbmt.org/activity.html [June 2005]). More details on the current indications for transplantation are available from the International Bone Marrow Transplant Registry, Center for International Blood and Marrow Transplant Research, Milwaukee, Wisconsin. See also Loberiza, "Report on the Art," slides 7 and 8.

79. Loberiza, "Report on State of the Art," slide 20; A. L. Lennard and G. H. Jackson, "Stem Cell Transplantation," *British Medical Journal* 321 (August 12, 2000): 433–37

80. Ibid., p. 434.

81. National Marrow Donor Program, "Disease Information" (www.marrow. org/patient/disease_info.html [June 2005]).

82. Fifteen percent of all allogenic transplants are now done in patients over age fifty, 2 percent in patients over age sixty. According to the International Bone Marrow Transplantation Registry, 20 percent of autograft recipients worldwide are over sixty, while virtually no allograft patients are this old. Loberiza, "Report on State of the Art," p. 8, slides 5–7.

83. For patients with chronic myeloid leukemia, for instance, outcomes for transplants from unrelated donors now approach those for transplants between siblings, although transplants from closely matched donors remain superior. Ibid., slides 11 and 12.

84. Ibid., slides 9, 10, and 19. For evidence on the increased use of unrelated donor allografts in Europe, see Alois Gratwohl and others, "Economics, Health Care Systems and Utilization of Haematopoietic Stem Cell Transplants in Europe," *British Journal of Haematology* 117, no. 2 (2002): 451–68.

85. Recent evidence suggests that the use of peripheral blood cells permits faster engraftment than use of bone marrow cells and may yield higher disease-free survival rates, particularly among allograft recipients with advanced blood cancers. Allografts that use peripheral blood cells are also marginally less expensive than allografts using bone marrow cells. William I. Bensinger and others, "Transplantation of Bone Marrow as Compared with Peripheral-Blood Cells from HLA-Identical Relatives in Patients with Hematologic Cancers," *New England Journal of Medicine* 344, no. 3 (2001): 175–81; C. L. Bennett and others, "Valuing Clinical Strategies Early in Development: A Cost Analysis of Allogeneic Peripheral Blood Stem Cell Transplantation," *Bone Marrow Transplantation* 24, no. 5 (1999): 555–60. See also Philip Jacobs and others, "Allogenic Stem Cell Transplantation: An Economic Comparison of Bone Marrow, Peripheral Blood, and Cord Blood Technologies," *International Journal of Technology Assessment in Health Care* 16, no. 3 (2000): 874–84.

86. In one recent study, 4 percent of patients with severe aplastic anemia who received transplants from matched relatives rejected their grafts. Rainer Storb and others, "Cyclophosphamide and Antithymocyte Globulin to Condition Patients with Aplastic Anemia for Allogeneic Marrow Transplantations: The Experience in Four Centers," *Biology of Blood and Marrow Transplantation* 7, no.1 (2001): 39-44.

87. Loberiza, "Report on State of the Art," slide 14. For all transplants registered with the International Bone Marrow Registry between 1996 and 2000, relapse accounted for 23 to 34 percent of deaths among allograft recipients and 78 percent among autograft recipients. The proportions of deaths related to infection were 5 percent for autografts, 17 percent for allografts with sibling donors, and 21 percent for allografts with unrelated donors.

88. Reem A. Abo-Zena and Mitchell E. Horwitz, "Immunomodulation in Stem-Cell Transplantation," *Current Opinion in Pharmacology* 2, no. 4, (2002): 452–57. A particular form of pneumonia affecting the lung's connective tissue caused less than 10 percent of deaths following transplants done from 1996 to 2000. Loberiza, "Report on State of the Art," slide 14. Mortality from graft-versus-host disease does not vary by whether or not a sibling or unrelated donor is used.

89. M. Arora and others, "Results of Autologous and Allogeneic Hematopoietic Cell Transplant Therapy for Multiple Myeloma," *Bone Marrow Transplantation* 35, no. 12 (2005): 1133–40. Predictably, death rates for autografts and allografts also correlate with disease stage at transplantation. Andrew Duncombe, "ABC of Clinical Haematology: Bone Marrow and Stem Cell Transplantation," *British Medical Journal* 314 (April 19, 1997): 1179. For charts of 100-day mortality by disease, see Loberiza, "Report on State of the Art," p. 9, slides 11, 12, and 13.

90. For a review of the clinical trials that prompted the drop in transplantation for breast cancer, see Karen H. Antman, "Overview of the Six Available Randomized Trials of High-Dose Chemotherapy with Blood or Marrow Transplant in Breast Cancer," *Journal of National Cancer Institute Monographs*, no. 30 (2001): 114–16. On trends in the use of transplantation for breast cancer patients in the United States, see Derek van Amerongen, "Insurance Payments for Bone Marrow Transplantation in Metastatic Breast Cancer," *New England Journal of Medicine*

342, no. 15 (2000): 1138–39. For trends in Europe, including the United Kingdom, see Gratwohl and others, "Economics," especially figure 5.

91. Loberiza, "Report on State of the Art" (rough estimates from slide 1).

92. John M. Goldman and Mary M. Horowitz, "The International Bone Marrow Transplant Registry," *International Journal of Hematology* 76, supplement 1 (August 2002): 393–97.

93. For data from the early 1980s, see Aaron and Schwartz, *Painful Prescription*, p. 53. During the early 1989–1991 period, the United Kingdom and the United States performed 0.82 and 0.81 allogenic transplants per 100,000 population per year, respectively. The majority of transplant recipients suffered from acute leukemia. Allografts were more common in France and Sweden, primarily because those countries were more likely than the United States and the United Kingdom to provide transplants to patients with diseases other than leukemia. George Silberman and others, "Availability and Appropriateness of Allogeneic Bone Marrow Transplantation for Chronic Myeloid Leukemia in 10 Countries," *New England Journal of Medicine* 331, no. 16 (1994): 1063–67. For recent comparisons, see U.K. data from the British Society of Blood and Marrow Transplantation, "Breakdown of All the U.K. Transplants for 2002" (www.bsbmt. org/activity.html#2002 [June 2005]). In 2002 the United States performed 17,160 procedures—5.95 transplants per 100,000 population—compared with 2,258 procedures in the United Kingdom—4.56 transplants per 100,000 population. See Richard Hauboldt and Nickolas Ortner, "2002 Organ and Tissue Transplant Costs and Discussion," Milliman USA Research Report (www.com/health/ pubs/HRR_07-2002.pdf [June 2005]). Patients with multiple myeloma and non-Hodgkin's lymphoma received over half of all stem cell transplants performed in North America in 2002, and virtually all of these patients served as their own stem cell donors. The data from the British Society of Blood and Marrow Transplantation show a similar picture for the United Kingdom. More detail on the current indications for transplantation is available from the International Bone Marrow Transplant Registry. See also Loberiza, "Report on State of the Art," slides 7 and 8.

94. U.S. data are from the Agency for Healthcare Research and Quality, "Healthcare Cost and Utilization Project" (www.ahrq.gov/data/hcup/ [July 2005]); see procedure codes 41.01–41.07. The data for the United Kingdom are from Department of Health, *NHS Reference Costs 2003* (London, 2004). The British data are for fiscal year 2003 and have been converted to U.S. dollars using a rate of $1.7 per pound, the then-prevailing exchange rate. Costs for pediatric stem cell transplants in the United Kingdom were generally similar to those for adults, except for a miscellaneous category that was twice as high.

95. Aaron and Schwartz, *Painful Prescription*, p. 52.

96. These estimates may be below actual spending. According to the Agency for Health Research and Quality, aggregate charges for stem cell transplants totaled $1.9 billion in 2001. Agency for Healthcare Research and Quality, "Healthcare Cost and Utilization Project." This estimate assumes that 10,710 transplants were performed in 2001. However, according to a report by the Milliman Corporation on organ and tissue transplant costs in the United States,

17,160 stem cell transplants were performed in 2002, and the number of procedures has tended to increase rapidly. See Hauboldt and Ortner, "2002 Organ and Tissue Transplant Costs." Expenditure on stem cell transplants in the United States in 1992 was taken from Ilana L. Westerman and Charles L. Bennett, "A Review of the Costs, Cost-Effectiveness and Third-Party Charges of Bone Marrow Transplantation," *Stem Cells* 14, no. 3 (1996): 312–19.

97. This estimate was calculated using the number of procedures performed in the U.K. in 2002 (British Society of Blood and Marrow Transplantation, "U.K. Transplants for 2002") multiplied by the estimated cost of the various types of procedures for 2002–03 from the British Department of Health, *NHS Reference Costs 2003*, table 2. The estimate is very crude because the cost categories do not strictly match the procedure categories. More specifically, it is assumed that the British did 353 allografts with bone marrow at $70,928 each; 471 allografts with peripheral blood stem cells at $74,221 each; 56 autografts with bone marrow at $53,291 per procedure; and 1,222 autografts with peripheral stem cells at $42,468 per procedure. This leads to a total cost estimate of $114,875,867.

98. In 2002, 4.56 transplants per 100,000 population were performed in the United Kingdom, well under the equivalent rate of 5.95 transplants per 100,000 in the United States in that year. U.K. data are from the British Society of Blood and Marrow Transplantation, "U.K. Transplants for 2002." U.S. data are from Hauboldt and Ortner, "2002 Organ and Tissue Transplant Costs."

99. Louise B. Russell, *Technology in Hospitals: Medical Advances and Their Diffusion* (Brookings, 1979), p. 41.

100. The first earmarked funds for intensive care units were made available in 1962. See Intensive Care Society, *Evolution of Intensive Care in the U.K.* (London, 2003), p. 4. A nationwide survey in Britain indicated that nine of every ten trusts had a "general ICU" in 1998, sometimes including intermediate and coronary care as well as intensive care beds. Audit Commission, *Critical to Success: The Place of Efficient and Effective Critical Care Services within the Acute Hospital* (London, 1999), p. 12. According to the Intensive Care Society, "During the 1970s and 80s the modern concept of critical illness developed. . . . It was often only one or two enthusiastic clinicians within a hospital who established and managed the intensive care unit." See Intensive Care Society, "Evolution of Intensive Care in the U.K." (www.ics.ac.uk/downloads/icshistory.pdf [June 2005]), p. 4.

101. The European Union of Medical Specialists defines intensive care as "continuous (that is, 24 hours) management including monitoring, diagnostics, support of failing vital functions, as well as the treatment of the underlying diseases." European Union of Medical Specialists (UEMS), *UEMS Compendium of Medical Specialists*, 1st ed. (London: Kensington Publications, 2000), pp. 142–43.

102. Intensive Care Society, *Standards for Intensive Care Units* (London, 1997), p. 14.

103. U.S. neonatal units tended to be larger than units for adults. The former had an average of twenty-one beds, while the latter averaged twelve. Data on the number of ICU beds per unit in the United States are from Jeffrey S. Groeger and others, "Descriptive Analysis of Critical Care Units in the United States," *Critical Care Medicine* 20, no. 6. (1992): 846–62. The distribution of intensive care patients by hospital size in the early 1990s was as follows: 10 percent in hospitals

with fewer than 100 beds, 40 percent in hospitals with 100 to 300 beds, 30 percent in hospitals with 300 to 500 beds, and 20 percent in hospitals with more than 500 beds. Bruce Gipe, "ICU Administration," in *Critical Care Medicine: Principles of Diagnosis and Management in the Adult*, 2nd ed., edited by Joseph E. Parrillo and R. Philip Dellinger (St. Louis, Mo.: Mosby, 2001), p. 1542. Data on intensive care beds in England in 1993 are from Alison Metcalfe and Kim McPherson, *Study of Provision of Intensive Care in England, 1993* (London: Department of Health, 1995), p. 8, and Audit Commission, *Critical to Success*, p. 17. Averages for other European nations are: Austria (10), Belgium (19), Denmark (14), France (11), Germany (12), Holland (10), Spain (14), Sweden (13), and Switzerland (14). David Edbrooke, Clare Hibbert, and Margaret Corcoran, *Review for the NHS Executive of Adult Critical Care Services: An International Perspective* (Sheffield, U.K.: Medical Economics and Research Centre, August 1999), p. 6.

104. Edbrooke, Hibbert, and Corcoran, *Review for the NHS*. If nurses work forty-hour weeks and are off 15 percent of the time for vacation, illness, or other reasons, the British ratio translates into one nurse for every 1.2 beds at any given moment.

105. Intensive Care Beds, England and the United States, 1982–2002

Units as indicated

ICU beds	1982[a]	1993[b]	2002
Number			
England	1,216–2,432	1,829–3,146	3,030
United States	59,698	92,792	85,203
As percent of all beds			
England	0.5–1.1	1.1–1.9	2.2
United States	5.9	10	10
Per 100,000 population			
England	2.6–5.2	3.8–6.5	6.1
United States	26	36	30
England as percent of United States	10–20	11–18	20

Sources: Robert A. Berenson, *Intensive Care Units (ICUs): Clinical Outcomes, Costs, and Decisionmaking,* Health Technology Case Study 28 (Washington, D.C.: Office of Technology Assessment, November 1984), p. 16; American Hospital Association (AHA), *Hospital Statistics 2003* (Chicago: Health Forum, 2003), p. 4; AHA, *Hospital Statistics 1994* (Chicago: Health Forum, 1994), pp. 234–41; U.K. Department of Health, *Shaping the Future NHS: Long Term Planning for Hospitals and Related Services* (London, 2000), p. 35; Department of Health, "January 2002 Census of Adult Critical Care" (www.dh.gov.uk [June 2005]); Metcalfe and McPherson, *Study of Provision of Intensive Care in England, 1993* (London: Department of Health, 1995).

a. The only hard number for 1982 is the U.S. bed count. Other numbers were derived on the assumption that the British had 10 to 20 percent the number of intensive care beds as the Americans on a population-adjusted basis in 1982.

b. The count of ICU beds in the United States for 1993 is an underestimate because it fails to capture a residual "other" category of intensive care, which is included in the 2002 bed count. In 2002 about 6,000 ICU beds fell into this category. Personal communication from Kim Garber, AHA, 2003. An adjusted 1993 bed count is available from AHA for $10–$30.

106. Russell, *Technology in Hospitals,* pp. 47–49. Noseworthy and Jacobs estimate that ICU beds cost seven times as much as regular beds. See Thomas W. Noseworthy and Philip Jacobs, "Economics of Critical Care," in *Principles in Critical Care,* edited by Jesse B. Hall and others (McGraw-Hill, 1998), p. 20. If this estimate were valid, ICU costs would account for just under half of all hospital costs.

107. Data on the costs of ICUs in the United Kingdom are from Audit Commission, *Critical to Success,* p. 18, and David Edbrooke and others, "The Development of a Method for Comparative Costing of Individual Intensive Care Units," *Anaesthesia* 54, no. 2 (1999): 110–20. Data on the total hospital spending budget are from Department of Health, *Departmental Report 2000–2001,* chaps. 3 and 11 (www.dh.gov.uk/PublicationsAndStatistics/Publications/Annual-Reports/fs/en [June 2005]).

108. Aaron and Schwartz, *Painful Prescription,* p. 96.

109. Ibid., p. 102.

110. Wight and Cohen, "Shortage of Organs."

Chapter Four

1. One of the primary motives for purchasing private insurance is the belief, often exaggerated, regarding average waiting times for NHS services. See chapter 2, note 44.

2. Waiting lists grew 31 percent between 1977 and 1979. Philip Wood, ed., *Challenge of Arthritis and Rheumatism: A Report on Problems and Progress in Health Care for Rheumatic Disorders* (London: Her Majesty's Stationery Office [HMSO], 1977), p. 48; and Working Party, Secretary of State for Social Services, *Orthopaedic Services: Waiting Time for Out-Patient Appointments and In-Patient Treatment* (London: HMSO, 1981), p. 4.

3. Waiting data for 1977 are from Working Party, *Orthopaedic Services,* p. 3. For 2003–04 waiting times, see Department of Health, "Hospital Waiting Times/List Statistics" (www.performance.doh.gov.uk/waitingtimes/index.htm [July 2005]). Average waiting times for 2002 are from Department of Health, *Hospital Episode Statistics 2001/2002* (www.hesonline.nhs.uk [July 2005]).

4. See "History of Total Hip Replacement" (www.thehipdoc.com/history.htm [June 2005]).

5. National Institute for Clinical Excellence, *Hip Prostheses Assessment Report* (March 2000), table 7; C. G. Moran and L. J. Tourret, "Recent Advancers: Orthopaedics," *British Medical Journal* 322 (April 14, 2001): 902.

6. John Charnley, the discoverer of polymethylmethacrylate, reported that well under 1 percent a year of the hips he replaced required surgery because of loosening. See A. J. Harrold, "Outlook for Hip Replacement," *British Medical Journal* 284 (January 16, 1982): 139. An earlier article reported a failure rate of 54 percent over five years for patients under thirty. Hugh P. Chandler, F. Timothy Reineck, and Richard L. Wixson, "A Five Year Review of Total Hip Replacement in Patients under 30—with Emphasis on Loosening," *Orthopedic Transactions* 3, no. 303 (1979).

7. Stephen Frankel and others, "Population Requirement for Primary Hip-Replacement Surgery: A Cross-Sectional Study," *Lancet* 353, no. 9161 (1999): 1304–09.

8. Henry J. Aaron and William B. Schwartz, *The Painful Prescription* (Brookings, 1984), p. 61.

9. Comptroller and Auditor General, *Hip Replacements: Getting It Right First Time*, HC 417 Session 1999-00 (London: National Audit Office, April 19, 2000), p. 44.

10. Angina may also result from other causes, particularly in women. These causes include narrowing of the aortic valve, anemia, and hyperthyroidism. See Texas Heart Institute, "Angina" (www.tmc.edu/thi/angina.html [June 2005]).

11. A heart attack can also result when a plaque deposit ruptures and the resulting fragments form a blockage. See Texas Heart Institute, "Heart Attack" (www.tmc.edu/thi/attack.html [June 2005]).

12. Data on first statin use from Jeremy Quirk, Mark Thornton, and Peter Kirkpatrick, "Fresh from the Pipeline: Rosuvastatin Calcium," *Nature Reviews* 2 (October 2003): 769–70. A new drug, torcetrapib, holds some promise of increasing high-density lipoprotein, so-called "good cholesterol." Alex Berenson, "Pfizer Stirs Concern with Plans to Sell Heart Drugs Only as Pair," *New York Times*, March 7, 2005, p. A1.

13. U.S. data are from American Heart Association, "Angioplasty and Cardiac Revascularization Statistics," *Heart and Stroke Encyclopedia* (www.americanheart.org/presenter.jhtml?identifier=4439 [June 2005]), and from the Agency for Healthcare Research and Quality, "Healthcare Cost and Utilization Project (HCUP)" (www.ahrq.gov/data/hcup [June 2005]). For U.K. data, see British Heart Foundation, "Coronary Heart Disease Statistics–2005" (www.heartstats.org/datapage.asp?id=5340 [July 6, 2005]), pp. 66–67.

14. The innovator was David C. Sabiston Jr. of the Johns Hopkins University. See Mani Sivasubramanian, "Coronary Artery Bypass Grafting—History and Technique" (www.heartdiseaseonline.com/aa/aa080397.htm [June 2005]).

15. L. Henry Edmunds, "Cardiopulmonary Bypass after 50 Years," *New England Journal of Medicine* 351, no. 16 (2004): 1603–06.

16. Personal communication from Alan Garber, Stanford University, March 2005. Mortality rates also vary with the patient's age and health. National Institutes of Health Consensus Development Conference, "Coronary Artery Bypass Surgery: Scientific and Clinical Aspects," *New England Journal of Medicine* 304 (March 12, 1981): 680–84. According to a U.S. Veterans Administration study, the four-year survival rates for patients with severe left main artery disease were 89 percent for surgically treated patients and 60 percent for medically treated ones. According to a European randomized study, the comparable survival rates for three-vessel disease were 89 percent and 67 percent, respectively. See Aaron and Schwartz, *Painful Prescription*.

17. Harold S. Luft and others, "Should Operations Be Regionalized? The Empirical Relation between Surgical Volume and Mortality," *New England Journal of Medicine* 310 (December 20, 1979): 1365. See also American Heart Association, *Heart Disease and Stroke: 2005 Update* (Dallas, Tex., 2005), p. 51.

18. Jeffrey W. Moses and others, "Sirolimus-Eluting Stents versus Standard Stents in Patients with Stenosis in a Native Coronary Artery," *New England Journal of Medicine* 349, no. 14 (2003): 1315–23.

19. Figures for 1982 from the National Center for Health Care Technology, *Technology Assessment Forum, Coronary Artery Bypass Surgery*, special report (Washington, June 23, 1981), pp. 1, 4, 8; Editorial, "Coronary Artery Bypass Surgery—Indications and Limitations," *Lancet* 2 (September 6, 1980): 511; and Gina Kolata, "Some Bypass Surgery Unnecessary," *Science* 222 (November 11, 1983): 605. In 2002, 515,000 CABG procedures were performed at an average of $60,853 per procedure, for a total cost of $31.3 billion. In 2002 the average costs of the various types of procedures included in 1,204,000 angioplasties ranged from $33,077 to $64,965, translating to a total of $42.7 billion. Total health care spending in 2002 was $1.6 trillion, and direct patient care costs, calculated as the sum of payments to hospitals and physicians, were $896 billion. For costs of CABG and angioplasty procedures, see Agency for Healthcare Research and Quality, "Healthcare Cost and Utilization Project" (www.ahrq.gov/data/hcup [July 2005]). Health spending data for 2002 are from Cathy Cowan and others, "National Health Expenditures, 2002," *Health Care Financing Review* 25, no. 4 (2004): 143–66.

20. Henning R. Andersen and others., "A Comparison of Coronary Angioplasty with Fibrinolytic Therapy in Acute Myocardial Infarction," *New England Journal of Medicine* 349, no. 8 (2003): 733–42.

21. The British estimate is from Gina Kolata, "Consensus on Bypass Surgery," *Science* 211 (January 2, 1981): 42–43. U.S. estimates are from Office of Technology Assessment, *The Implications of Cost Effectiveness Analysis of Medical Technology,* Background Paper 4: *The Management of Health Care Technology in Ten Countries* (Washington, 1980), p. 212.

22. U.S. treatment numbers used to derive these rates come from American Heart Association, "Angioplasty and Cardiac Revascularization Statistics," and from Agency for Healthcare Research and Quality, "Healthcare Cost and Utilization Project." U.K. treatment numbers are from British Heart Foundation, "Coronary Heart Disease Statistics—2005." U.S. population data used to derive these rates are from Bureau of the Census, "Table NA-EST2002-01–National Population Estimates: April 1, 2000 to July 1, 2002" (www.census.gov/popest/archives/2000s/vintage_2002/NA-EST2002-01.html [July 2005]). U.K. population data are from Office of National Statistics, "T 01: United Kingdom; Estimated Resident Population by Single Year of Age and Sex; Revised in Light of the Local Authority Population Studies; Mid-2002 Population Estimates" (www.statistics.gov.uk/StatBase/ssdataset.asp?vlnk=8535&Pos=9&ColRank=1&Rank=272 [July 2005]).

23. See British Heart Foundation, "Factfile 05/2004: Drug Eluting Stents" (www.bhf.org.uk/professionals/uploaded/may04.pdf [June 2005]), citing data from British Cardiovascular Intervention Society Audit Returns, "Adult Interventional Procedures," PowerPoint presentation, slide 53 (www.cardiology.co.uk/bcis/audit_data_2002.ppt [June 2005]).

24. Ernst R. Berndt and others, "Medical Care Prices and Output," in *Handbook*

of Health Economics, vol. 1A, edited by Anthony J. Culyer and Joseph P. Newhouse (New York: Elsevier, 2000), pp. 119–80.

25. British Heart Foundation, "International Comparisons in Mortality" (www.heartstats.org/datapage.asp?id=744 [June 2005]).

26. Lee Goldman and E. Francis Cook, "The Decline in Ischemic Heart Disease Mortality Rates: An Analysis of the Comparative Effects of Medical Interventions and Changes in Lifestyle," *Annals of Internal Medicine* 101, no. 6 (1984): 825–36.

27. Personal communication from David Cutler, Harvard University, November 11, 2004.

28. Heidenreich and McClellan attributed 90 percent of the reduction from 1975 to 1995 in mortality in the thirty days after a heart attack to the increasing use of aspirin, clot-busting drugs, angioplasty, beta-blockers, ACE (angiotensin-converting enzyme) inhibitors, and other medical interventions. See Paul Heidenreich and Mark McClellan, "Trends in Treatment and Outcomes for Acute Myocardial Infarction: 1975–1995," *American Journal of Medicine* 110, no. 3 (2001): 165–74. McClellan and Newhouse found that surgical procedures reduced by 27 percent the probability of a patient's death within two years after a heart attack. Mark McClellan and Joseph P. Newhouse, "The Marginal Cost-Effectiveness of Medical Technology: A Panel Instrumental-Variables Approach," *Journal of Econometrics* 77, no. 1 (1997): 39–64.

29. Such screening remains far from complete. The National Health and Nutrition Examination Survey (NHANES) reported that 65.4 percent of the U.S. population over age sixty has hypertension, but only 27.4 percent of this group have their condition controlled. Ihab Hajjar and Theodore A. Kotchen, "Trends in Prevalence, Awareness, Treatment and Control of Hypertension in the United States, 1988–2000," *Journal of the American Medical Association* 290, no. 2 (2003): 199–206, as cited in Bruce Pyenson and others, *Controlling Hypertension among Medicare Beneficiaries: Saving Lives without Additional Cost* (Brookfield, Wisc.: Milliman Consultants and Actuaries, September, 2004), p. 3.

30. American Cancer Society, "Updated Breast Cancer Screening Guidelines Released" (www.cancer.org/docroot/NWS/content/NWS_1_1x_Updated_Breast_Cancer_Screening_Guidelines_Released.asp [May 15, 2003]).

31. British standards for controlling blood pressure were set at 150/90 until 2004 and then were lowered to 140/90. According to U.S. standards, patients were hypertensive if their blood pressure was 140/90 or above, except that the recommended threshold for patients with chronic kidney disease or diabetes was 130/80 or less. See National High Blood Pressure Education Program, *The Seventh Report of the Joint National Committee on Prevention, Detection, Evaluation, and Treatment of High Blood Pressure* (www.nhlbi.nih.gov/guidelines/hypertension/express.pdf [December 2003]).

32. Evidence from a recent study indicated that high doses of atorvastatin (Lipitor), sufficient to reduce low-density lipoprotein (LDL) to mean levels of 77 milligrams per deciliter versus 100 milligrams per deciliter, reduced major cardiovascular events and stroke. Peggy Peck, "High-Dose Statins Reduce Cardiac Risk, Study Says," *AMNews.COM*, April 4, 2005 (www.ama-assn.org/amednews/2005/04/04/hlsb0404.htm).

33. Aaron and Schwartz, *Painful Prescription*, pp. 64–65.

34. "Coronary Artery Bypass Surgery," p. 511. Or, as one British general practitioner put it, "There are very few cases where coronary artery surgery is mandatory as an emergency. The typical case is treated to the full medically. Patients are asked to stop smoking. They are asked to lose weight. They are put on all of the different drugs. If they are still disabled then, or if it looks like it's a certain type of coronary artery disease, then one would refer them to a consultant a bit more quickly. And they would be seen by the consultant more promptly if I asked him to try to do it this week. Then the cardiologist decides what to do, whether or not to do arteriography, and if surgery is necessary, it would usually be done in one to four months."

35. National Institutes of Health Consensus Development Conference, "Coronary Artery Bypass Surgery: Scientific and Clinical Aspects," *New England Journal of Medicine* 304 (March 12, 1981): 680.

36. Kolata, "Consensus on Bypass Surgery." A British internist in the early 1980s affirmed these differences between U.S. and British attitudes in a letter: "I have been much involved with patients who have been investigated and subjected to surgery in the U.S.A., including some of the best medical centers there, and I have seen quite a lot of U.S. medicine first hand. What impresses me is that in comparison with the U.K., it seems very seldom that the U.S. physician ever states that there is no surgery that would help, no drug that is advantageous, and no further investigation that is required. There seems to be an irresistible urge always to do something, even though in many cases the doctor concerned must realize that there is no possibility of benefit."

Finally, another American cardiologist wrote, "That there are fundamental differences in the personality structure of an Englishman versus an American seems to be well established throughout contemporary literature and the cartoons of our time. One has a 'stiff upper lip,' the other is flamboyant to the point of 'wearing it on his sleeve.' One, genteel and reserved; the other, macho. . . . The American demands surgery and . . . wants the consolation of having done everything possible. The Englishman tends to be more philosophical in approach and perhaps demands less."

37. Angela M. Tod and others, "Barriers to Uptake of Services for Coronary Heart Disease: Qualitative Study," *British Medical Journal* 323 (July 28, 2001): 214.

38. In December of 2004, the American Medical Association listed 1,083 specialists in cardiovascular disease in New Jersey. In 2004 the NHS employed 685 cardiologists. For U.S. data, see American Medical Association, "Physician-Related Data Resources" (www.ama-assn.org/cgi-bin/sserver/datalist.cgi?State= NJ [January 2005]); for data for the United Kingdom, see British Heart Foundation, "BHF Coronary Heart Disease Statistics 2004" (www.bhf.org.uk/professionals/index.asp?SecID=15&secondlevel=519 [June 2005]).

39. Manish Gandhi, Fiona Lampe, and David Wood, "Management of Angina Pectoris in General Practice: A Questionnaire Survey of General Practitioners," *British Journal of General Practice* 45, no. 390 (1995): 11–13. Richard Martin and others, "Population Need for Coronary Revascularisation: Are National Targets for England Credible?" *Heart* 88, no. 6 (2002): 627–33.

40. John K. Inman, "What a General Practitioner Wants from a Referral Service for Suspected Angina," in *Management of Stable Angina*, edited by David de Bono and Anthony Hopkins (London: Royal College of Physicians, 1994), pp. 38–44.

41. Ibid.

42. In 2000-01 the proportion of the population admitted as surgical inpatients was more than three times as high in the United States as in England. U.S. data are from *OECD Health Data 2002*, 4th ed. Data for England are from Department of Health, *Hospital Episode Statistics 2000/01*, "Table 4. Main Operations—Summary" (www.hesonline.nhs.uk [July 2005]). In addition, back surgery is performed five times as often in the United States as in England and Wales, and surgical biopsies for breast cancer screening are performed at rates twice as high in the United States as in the United Kingdom. D. C. Cherkin and others, "An International Comparison of Back Surgery Rates," *Spine* 19, no. 11 (1994): 1201-6; Rebecca Smith-Bindman and others, "Comparison of Screening Mammography in the United States and the United Kingdom," *Journal of the American Medical Association* 290, no. 16 (2003): 2129–37. For an early comparison of surgery rates, see John P. Bunker, "Surgical Manpower: A Comparison of Operations and Surgeons in the United States and in England and Wales," *New England Journal of Medicine* 282 (January 15, 1970): 135–44.

43. Michael G. Chernew, Gautam Gowrisankaran, and A. Mark Frederick, "Payer Type and the Returns to Bypass Surgery: Evidence from Hospital Entry Behavior," *Journal of Health Economics* 21, no. 3 (2002): 451–74.

44. The United States uses angiography, angioplasty, and CABG at far higher rates than does Canada but achieves medical results that are only slightly better three months after a heart attack and not at all better after one year. Jack V. Tu and others, "Use of Cardiac Procedures and Outcomes in Elderly Patients with Myocardial Infarction in the United States and Canada," *New England Journal of Medicine* 336, no. 21 (1997):1500–05.

45. Personal communications with Howard Glennerster, London School of Economics (emeritus), 2003–04. For details on terms and conditions of the consultants' contracts, see Department of Health, "Terms and Conditions—Consultants (England) 2003" (www.dh.gov.uk/assetRoot/04/06/99/07/04069907.pdf [June 2005]).

46. Gautam Gowrisankaran, "Productivity in Heart Attack Treatments," *Federal Reserve Bank of San Francisco Economic Letter*, no. 2002-20 (July 5, 2002): 1–3.

Chapter Five

1. The proportion of cases in which the condition is present and is correctly identified by the test is known as the test's *sensitivity*. The proportion of the cases in which the test correctly shows that the condition is not present is known as its *specificity*.

2. A new test for colon cancer using DNA illustrates the pitfalls of improved accuracy. This test is markedly more sensitive than the traditional test based on

occult blood in stool samples. However, its specificity is not markedly higher than the older test. The new test is many times more costly than the old. Furthermore, the incidence of colon cancer is so low that the number of false positives will vastly exceed the number of true positives. Because DNA tests are so widely trusted, the potential for greatly increased costs and overtreatment led one physician to urge that the new test not be used. Steven H. Woolf, "A Smarter Strategy?—Reflections on Fecal DNA Screening for Colorectal Cancer," *New England Journal of Medicine* 351, no. 26 (2004): 2755–58.

3. Detailed information on the technology and practice of CT scanning is available on the Internet. See, for example, Hans Dieter Nagel, "Multislice CT Technology" (www.multislice-ct.com/www [July 2005]); *Wikipedia*, "Computed Axial Tomography" (en.wikipedia.org/wiki/computed_axial_tomography [June 2005]); National Cancer Institute, "Cancer Facts: Computed Tomography (CT): Questions and Answers" (cis.nci.nih.gov/fact/5_2.htm [September 2003]).

4. Nagel, "Multislice," p. 1; Siemens, "Siemens Releases the World's First Clinical Images from 64-Slice CT Scanner," press release, May 10, 2004. Available at their U.S. website: www.medical.siemens.com/webapp/wcs/stores/servlet/StoreCatalogDisplay?storeId=10001&catalogId=-1&langId=-1 [June 2005].

5. Imaginis, "Computed Tomography Imaging" (www.imaginis.com/ct-scan/spiral.asp [May 2004]).

6. Nagel, "Multislice," p. 6.

7. CT scans do not show the presence of coronary disease when disease is absent (high specificity), but they sometimes fail to identify actual disease (low sensitivity). Thus CT scans can be used instead of invasive angiography to confirm the results of another test that suggests disease is not present, but they cannot now be relied on to detect disease. Interview with Dr. Christopher Putman, Fairfax Hospital, Fairfax, Virginia, July 6, 2004.

8. Gina Kolata, "Consensus on CT Scans," *Science* 214 (December 18, 1981): 1327–28; and National Institutes of Health Consensus Program, "Computed Tomographic Scanning of the Brain," *NIH Consensus Statement* 4, no. 2 (November 4–6, 1981): 1–7.

9. In 2004 dollars the cost of a new single-slice scanner in 1980 was more than $1.4 million, and a used machine cost just over $200,000.

10. Personal communication from Bill Yovik, Barrington Medical Imaging (a seller of used and refurbished machines), Lake Barrington, Illinois, May 2004.

11. Harvey L. Nisenbaum and others, "The Costs of CT Procedures in an Academic Radiology Department Determined by an Activity-Based Costing (ABC) Method," *Journal of Computer Assisted Tomography* 24, no. 5 (2000): 813–23; William W. Mayo-Smith and others, "Transportable versus Fixed Platform CT Scanners: Comparison of Costs," *Radiology* 226, no.1 (2003): 63–68; Sanjay Saini and others, "Technical Cost of CT Examinations," *Radiology* 218, no.1 (2001): 172–75; Sanjay Saini, "Technical Cost of Radiologic Examinations: Analysis across Imaging Modalities," *Radiology* 216, no. 1 (2000): 269–72.

12. See Henry J. Aaron and William B. Schwartz, *The Painful Prescription* (Brookings, 1984), p. 70.

13. Nisenbaum and others, "Costs of CT Procedures."

14. Mayo-Smith and others, "Transportable versus Fixed Platform CT." Excluding overhead, the per exam cost is $75 when volume is high, and $112 when volume is low. A low-volume machine is taken to be one that is operational Monday through Friday, eight hours a day. The high-volume machine is taken to be operational seven days a week, twenty-four hours a day (in an emergency room, for instance).

15. Department of Health, *Reference Costs 2001* (London, 2002). Conversion to dollars is based on an exchange rate of £0.69 per U.S. dollar. U.S. Federal Reserve, "Foreign Exchange Rates," January 2, 2002 (www.federalreserve.gov/releases/g5a/20020102/ [June 2005]).

16. Compare the report of the Department of Health and Social Services, "Whole Body CT Scanners in England and Wales" (London, 1981), with Ronald G. Evens and R. Gilbert Jost, "Economic Analysis of Body Computed Tomography Units Including Data on Utilization," *Radiology* 127, no. 1 (1978): 151–57.

17. Data for 1980 come from Office of Technology Assessment, *Policy Implications of the CT Scanner* (Washington, 1981), pp. 15–17; Department of Health and Social Services, "Whole Body CT Scanners," p. 1. Data for 2001 come from a personal communication from Ken Bokina, IMV Medical Diagnostics Division for the United States, May 2004, and from Organization for Economic Cooperation and Development (OECD), *OECD Health Data 2002*, 4th ed. (Paris, 2002); Health Forum, *Hospital Statistics* 2004 (Chicago: American Hospital Association, 2003), p. 156–8; European Coordination Committee of the Radiological and Electromedical Industries, *Age Profile Medical Devices*, 3rd ed. (Frankfurt, February 2003), p. 12. The OECD source reports many fewer CT scanners than Bokina does, apparently because the OECD reports the number of hospitals with scanners, although many scanners are outside hospitals and many hospitals have two or more scanners. The OECD reports that Japan has nearly three times as many scanners per million population as the United States; Bokina's estimates indicate that the United States has slightly more scanners than any other listed country.

18. Other estimates put the number of scans far higher or lower. According to the Health Care Utilization Project of the Agency for Healthcare Research and Quality, a total of 875,214 scans were performed on inpatients of U.S. hospitals. Since the majority of scans are performed either on hospital outpatients or in freestanding facilities, this number is doubtlessly a small fraction of the total. The United Nations estimated that the annual average number of scans in the United States was 91,000 per million from 1991 through 1996. See United Nations Scientific Committee on the Effects of Atomic Radiation, *Sources and Effects of Ionizing Radiation: UNSCEAR 2000 Report to the General Assembly*, vol. 1, table 12 (www.unscear.org/reports/2000_1.html [July 2005]). Two other studies reached similar estimates: Fred A. Mettler and others, "CT Scanning: Patterns of Use and Dose," *Journal of Radiological Protection* 20 (2000): 355–56; Solucient, *Top Growth Areas in Outpatient Market* (Evanston, Ill., 2001), p. 5. Another recently published study suggests that the number of CT scans performed in American hospitals was more than twice as high—200,000 scans per million in 2001. See B. F. Wall, "What Needs to Be Done about Reducing Patient Doses

from CT? The North American Approach," *British Journal of Radiology* 76, no. 911a (2003): 763–65.

19. Department of Health, "Hospital Activity Statistics: Imaging and Radio-diagnostics, NHS Organisations in England, 2000–01" (www.performance.doh. gov.uk/hospitalactivity/data_requests/imaging_and_radiodiagnostics.htm [June 2005]).

20. The article by Wall cited in note 18 suggests that the cross-national gap in the availability of computed tomography is much larger than 4 to 1. He states that the rate of scans performed on American patients in 2000–01 was seven times higher than the corresponding U.K. rate in 2003. Unfortunately, the author does not specify the source of his data. A leading manufacturer of CT scanners reported that in 2003 the number of scanners per million was 10.5 in France, 28.6 in Germany, 28.8 in the United States, 24.3 in Italy, 16.7 in Spain, and 7.1 in the United Kingdom. Statistics reported in personal communication from Dr. Janet Husband, president, Royal College of Radiologists, London, 2004.

21. National Institutes of Health, "Computed Tomographic Scanning."

22. Care must be taken to make sure that the body of the MRI subject does not contain metal, such as implants or staples used during some surgery, because of possible physical injury. Some concern remains about the cellular effects of extremely powerful magnetic fields that are stronger than those used in MRI examinations on humans.

23. Ensil International Corporation, "The History of MRI" (www.ensil.com/ international/Database/database.html [June 2005]).

24. The U.S. data are from Ken Bokina, IMV Medical Diagnostics Division. The data for the United Kingdom are from the European Coordination Committee, *Age Profile Medical Devices*, p. 13. A leading manufacturer of MRI machines reports similar statistics for 2003: United Kingdom, 5.5 per million population; United States, 21.7; Germany, 14.6; and France, only 3.8. Personal communication from Dr. Janet Husband.

An estimated 18 million MRI procedures were performed in the United States in 2001, just under one-third of the worldwide total. Personal communication from Ken Bokina. This private estimate exceeds totals used in the cost estimates reported in the following section.

25. In 1993 and 1995, 46.5 and 44.6 percent of MRI magnets, respectively, were located outside hospitals, according to Laurence C. Baker, "Managed Care and Technology Adoption in Health Care: Evidence from Magnetic Resonance Imaging," *Journal of Health Economics* 20, no. 3 (2001):395–421. In 2001, 48.2 percent of MRI machines were outside hospitals.

26. For data on England, see Department of Health, "Hospital Activity Statistics." U.S. data are from Ken Bokina, personal communication.

27. Personnel, maintenance, insurance, utilities, and disposable supplies cost an estimated $420,000 per machine in 1995 in the United States for facilities performing 2,500 procedures. Given a five-year depreciable life for a machine, plus operating costs (adjusted for general inflation since 1995), estimated total costs for performing 2,500 procedures in 2004 were approximately $800,000 a year. Applying this cost to the 4,970 MRI scanners in the United States yields the

text estimate. Baker, "Managed Care," p. 415, citing Robert A. Bell, "Economics of MRI Technology," *Journal of Magnetic Resonance Imaging* 6, no. 1 (1996): 10–25.

28. Two studies relate to the cost of MRI in Bristol: J. L. Thomson, "Experiences at the New Magnetic Resonance Imaging Centre at Bristol," *British Journal of Radiology* 62, no. 734 (1989): 134–37; and J. L. Thomson, A. Case, and R. Williams, "Further Experience at the Bristol Centre, Following the Installation of a Second MRI Unit," *British Journal of Radiology* 66, no. 786 (1993): 493–96. Two others relate to costs of one facility in Coventry: J. Fletcher and others, "The Cost of MRI: Changes in Costs 1989–1996," *British Journal of Radiology* 72, no. 857 (1999): 432–37; and A. K. Szczepura, J. Fletcher, and J. D. Fitz-Patrick, "Cost Effectiveness of Magnetic Resonance Imaging in the Neurosciences," *British Medical Journal* 303 (December 7, 1991): 1435–39.

29. The Department of Health estimated the average "procedural cost" (operating costs plus estimated depreciation) of MRI exams in NHS hospitals at £286 ($407) in 2001. An estimated 632,594 MRI exams were performed in those hospitals. Department of Health, "Hospital Activity Statistics"; and Department of Health, *Reference Costs 2001.* Conversion to dollars based on an exchange rate of £0.69 per U.S. dollar. U.S. Federal Reserve, "Foreign Exchange Rates," January 2, 2002 (www.federalreserve.gov/releases/g5a/ 20020102/ [June 2005]).

30. See Aaron and Schwartz, *Painful Prescription*, p. 72.

31. Personal communication from Dr. Janet Husband.

32. Notes from interviews at INOVA-Fairfax Hospital, radiology department, Fairfax, Virginia, 2004. The former dean of one of the largest and most prestigious medical schools in the nation jokingly suggested that he sometimes thought that the MRI machine should be placed at the entrance to the emergency room, so that all patients who are admitted would routinely be scanned as they enter.

33. R. L. Harrison and others, "Vetting Requests for Body Computed Tomography," *European Radiology* 10, no. 6 (2000): 1015–18.

34. This six-stage approach to evaluation is based on methods applied by the U.S. Agency for Healthcare Research and Quality, as described by Athina Tatsioni and others, "Challenges in Systematic Reviews of Diagnostic Technologies," *Annals of Internal Medicine* 142, no. 12 (2005): 1048–55. This paper, in turn, applies analytical methods developed in earlier work. See John R. Thornbury, Denis G. Fryback, and Ward Edwards, "Likelihood Ratios as a Measure of the Diagnostic Usefulness of Excretory Urogram Information," *Radiology* 114, no.3 (1975): 561–65; Barbara J. McNeil and S. James Adelstein, "Determining the Value of Diagnostic and Screening Tests," *Journal of Nuclear Medicine* 17, no. 6 (1976): 439–48; Harvey V. Fineberg, Roger Bauman, and Martha Sosman, "Computerized Cranial Tomography: Effect on Diagnostic and Therapeutic Plans," *Journal of the American Medical Association* 238, no. 3 (1977): 224–27.

35. A. Wright and R. Bradford, "Fortnightly Review: Management of Acoustic Neuroma," *British Medical Journal* 311 (October 28, 1995): 1141–44.

36. Various British physicians speculate that U.S. physicians may be motivated both by the ready availability of MRI machines and concern about malpractice litigation.

37. Budget figures from Department of Health, "Departmental Report 2004" (www.dh.gov.uk/PublicationsAndStatistics/Publications/AnnualReports/fs/en [June 2005]).

Chapter Six

1. Some analysts have argued that health care markets will produce efficient outcomes if purchasers face the full cost of insurance. See, for example, Clark Havighurst and Barak D. Richman, "Distributive Injustice(s) in American Health Care," working paper 27, prepared for the American Law and Economics Association Fifteenth Annual Meeting, New York University, May 6–7, 2005. For this argument to be compelling, patients would have to enter into contracts far more detailed than any commonly written and make rational choices about matters concerning which they are almost entirely ignorant. Furthermore, one would have to believe that sick individuals should and will accept contractual terms they agreed to when healthy and that if preferences change between these two states, the preferences of the "healthy" person should override those of the "sick" one. This view is legally naive, contradicted by psychological research, and morally dubious.

2. This pattern shows up in comparisons across countries at a point in time and in particular countries over time. See chapter 1, note 9. Reinhardt, Hussey, and Anderson report a regression of total per capita health care spending on per capita GDP that yields an income elasticity of 1.36, based on cross-national data for 2001, for countries in the Organization for Economic Cooperation and Development. See Uwe Reinhardt, Peter Hussey, and Gerard Anderson, "U.S. Health Care Spending in an International Context," *Health Affairs* 23, no. 1 (2004): 10. Gerdtham and Jonsson suggest that income elasticities may in fact be nearer to 1.0. See Ulf-G. Gerdtham and Bengt Jonsson, "International Comparisons of Health Expenditure: Theory, Data, and Econometric Analysis," in *Handbook of Health Economics*, vol. 1A, edited by Anthony Culyer and Joseph Newhouse (New York: Elsevier, 2000), pp. 11–53. Actual per capita health care spending in the United States in 2001 was $4,887, which exceeded by 42 percent the $3,435 implied by the equation reported in Reinhardt, Hussey, and Anderson.

3. For comparison of physician pay, see chapter 2, note 54.

4. Many analysts distinguish questions of efficiency from issues of distribution. For many purposes this distinction is useful. In the case of health care, questions of efficient resource allocation and fair distribution are inextricably linked. For that reason, issues of distribution are just one part of the decision on how health care resources should be efficiently used.

5. Kevin Murphy and Robert Topel, eds., *Measuring the Gains from Medical Research: An Economic Approach* (University of Chicago Press, 2003); David M. Cutler and Mark McClellan, "Is Technological Change in Medicine Worth It?" *Health Affairs* 20, no. 5 (2001): 11–29; Ernst Berndt and others, "Medical Care Prices and Output," in *Handbook of Health Economics*, edited by Culyer and Newhouse, pp. 119–80.

6. Cutler and McClellan, "Is Technological Change in Medicine Worth It?"; Jonathan Skinner and John Wennberg, "How Much Is Enough? Efficiency and Medicare Spending in the Last Six Months of Life," in *The Changing Hospital Industry: Comparing Not-for-Profit and For-Profit Institutions*, edited by David Cutler (University of Chicago Press, 2000). More generally, see "The Dartmouth Atlas of Health Care 1999" (www.dartmouthatlas.org/atlaslinks/99atlas.php [June 2005]).

7. Fuchs and Garber's analogy of car insurance to health insurance, presented in chapter 1, suggests that health insurance distorts medical research, leading to quality and cost that are both probably higher than optimal, but the outcome may well be advances in technology worth far more than their total cost.

8. In the case of medical interventions, risk may not always be aversive. A procedure that offers a chance of complete recovery or death may be preferred to one that offers a certain prospect of impaired or pain-ridden existence, as long as the value attached to survival is not infinite.

9. If any of these efficiency conditions is not satisfied, benefit curves might not indicate how additional health care spending or cutbacks should be distributed. Inefficiency would mean that care was *not* being offered that was more beneficial than some care that *was* provided. Even if some actual outlays for a particular service were not worth what they cost, it might be rational to increase spending to fill gaps in the provision of that service.

10. The text ignores a complication of great practical importance. What constitutes the cost of a procedure is often far from clear. Procedures that require costly capital equipment, for example, may require a large expenditure to provide the service initially. But additional patients can be served at modest cost until the capacity of the machine is reached or until the machine has to be run for more than one normal work shift. In such situations the average cost of a procedure is far above the marginal cost of serving one more person, at least until the machine becomes congested.

11. Alan Williams, "Efficiency and Welfare," in *Providing for the Health Services*, edited by Douglas Black and G. P. Thomas (London: Croom Helm, 1978), pp. 31–32.

12. Psychologists challenge the assumption, so fundamental to welfare economics, that individuals have well-ordered preferences among commodities. Psychological research suggests, rather, that preferences are strongly dependent on the external context in which they are elicited and on the internal visceral state of the individual. Daniel Kahneman, Ilana Ritov, and David Schkade, "Economic Preferences or Attitude Expressions? An Analysis of Dollar Responses to Public Issues," *Journal of Risk and Uncertainty* 19 (December 1999): 203–352; George Loewenstein, "Out of Control: Visceral Influences on Behavior," *Organizational Behavior and Human Decision Processes* 65, no. 3 (1996): 272–92; Lee Ross and Richard E. Nisbett, *The Person and the Situation: Perspectives of Social Psychology* (New York: McGraw-Hill, 1991).

13. Bureau of Labor Statistics, "Comparative Real Gross Domestic Product per Capita and per Employed Person, Fourteen Countries, 1960–2003," July 26, 2004 (www.bls.gov/fls/flsgdp.pdf [June 2005]).

14. Data on United Kingdom earnings from Office of National Statistics, "Labour Market—New Earnings Survey 2003. United Kingdom: Streamlined and Summary Analyses; Description of the Survey" (www.statistics.gov.uk/downloads/theme_labour/NES2003_UK/NES2003_UK.pdf [July 2005]); U.S. data from Bureau of Labor Statistics, "2002 National Occupational Employment and Wage Estimates: Healthcare Practitioner and Technical Occupations" (www.bls.gov/oes/2002/oes_29he.htm [June 2005]) .

15. British Heart Foundation Statistics Database, "Age-Standardised Death Rates per 100,000 Population from CHD, Men, 1968–2001, Selected Countries, the World," and "Age-Standardised Death Rates per 100,000 Population from CHD, Women, 1968–2001, Selected Countries, the World" (www.heartstats.org [July 2005]).

16. While U.S. cancer mortality rates remain below those in the United Kingdom, the gap has narrowed significantly in recent decades. In 1979 the rate of deaths from cancer per 100,000 population was 30 points higher in the United Kingdom than in the United States; by 2001 that gap had narrowed to just under 10 points. See Organization for Economic Cooperation and Development, *OECD Health Data 2002,* 4th ed. (Paris, 2002).

17. U.K. population data from Office of National Statistics, "Table 12j: Mid-2000 Population Estimates; Quinary Age Groups and Sex for Health Areas in England and Wales; Estimated Resident Population Revised in Light of the Local Authority Population Studies" (www.statistics.gov.uk/statbase/ssdataset.asp?vlnk=8630&More=Y [June 2005]). U.S. data from Bureau of the Census, "QT-P1. Age Groups and Sex: 2000" (factfinder.census.gov/home/saff/main.html?_lang=en [June 2005]).

Chapter Seven

1. Alan Williams, "Efficiency and Welfare," in *Providing for the Health Services,* edited by Douglas Black and G. P. Thomas (London: Croom Helm, 1978), pp. 31–32.

2. If cost containment were to be approached through some method of cost-sharing rather than through revenue limits, these factors would likely play a different role, as indicated in the next chapter.

3. See Henry J. Aaron and William B. Schwartz, *The Painful Prescription* (Brookings, 1984), p. 90. The numbers have been converted from 1982 to 2004 prices, using the GDP deflator for health care.

4. Figures for 1980s from Aaron and Schwartz, *Painful Prescription,* p. 39. For recent estimates for the United Kingdom, see Christine Lee, Caroline Sabin, and Alexander Miners, "High Cost, Low Volume Care: The Case of Haemophilia," *British Medical Journal* 315 (October 1997): 962–63; for recent estimates for the United States, see National Hemophilia Foundation, "Financial and Insurance Issues" (www.hemophilia.org/bdi/bdi_issues.htm [June 2005]).

5. Henning R. Andersen and others, "A Comparison of Coronary Angioplasty with Fibrinolytic Therapy in Acute Myocardial Infarction," *New England Journal of Medicine* 349, no. 8 (2003): 733–42.

6. The first issue of *The Journal of Vascular and Interventional Radiology* was published in 1990.

7. For British data, see House of Commons, Treasury and Civil Service Committee, *Budget and the Government's Expenditure Plans, 1980–81 to 1983–84* (London: Her Majesty's Stationery Office, 1980), p. 104. For U.S. data, see Charles R. Fisher, "Differences by Age Groups in Health Care Spending," *Health Care Financing Review* 1 (Spring 1980): 81. Because the programs covered in the two sources are so different, the numbers in the text are approximations.

8. A strong argument can be made for the ethical imperative of allocating limited health resources to the young. For an example of such an argument made with respect to evaluating government regulatory interventions, see Cass R. Sunstein, "Lives, Life-Years, and Willingness to Pay," Working Paper 03-5 (AEI-Brookings Joint Center for Regulatory Studies, June 2003).

9. Aaron and Schwartz, *Painful Prescription*, p. 102.

10. Authors' interviews.

11. Organization for Economic Cooperation and Development, *OECD Health Data 2002*, 4th ed. (Paris, 2002).

12. Aaron and Schwartz, *Painful Prescription*, p. 107.

13. Office of Health Economics, *Hip Replacement and the NHS* (London: White Crescent Press, 1982).

14. For data for the United States, see "Dartmouth Atlas of Health Care, 2004" (www.dartmouthatlas.org [July 2005]). For the United Kingdom, see Department of Health, *Independent Inquiry into Inequalities in Health (Acheson Report)* (London: Her Majesty's Stationery Office, 1998).

15. Public Citizen, "Quick Facts on Medical Malpractice Issues" (www.citizen.org/congress/civjus/medmal/articles.cfm?ID=9125 [June 2005]).

16. National Health Service Litigation Authority, "The NHS Litigation Authority. Factsheet 1: Background Information" (www.nhsla.com/home.htm [June 2005]).

17. *Bolam* v. *Friern Hospital Management Committee* [1957] 2 All E.R. 118, as quoted in Michael A. Jones, *Medical Negligence*, 3rd ed. (London: Sweet and Maxwell, 2003).

18. Ibid.

19. The first case under these rules was decided by the House of Lords in November 1997. See Clare Dyer, "Medical Decisions Must Be Logically Defensible," *British Medical Journal* 315 (November 22, 1997): 1327–32.

20. Reportedly, some lawyers were unwilling to use the conditional fee system if the legal aid system guaranteed them payment. See Caroline Richmond, "Cost of Malpractice Protection on Rise in U.K., Too," *Canadian Medical Association Journal* 157, no. 7 (1997): 940–41; Anthony Barton, "Medical Litigation, Who Benefits?" *British Medical Journal* 322 (May 12, 2001): 1189.

21. Roger Dobson, "Legally Aided Medical Negligence Cases Fall Sharply," *British Medical Journal* 322 (April 28, 2001): 1018. See also Jones, *Medical Negligence*.

22. See "1,000 Kidney Patients Die Because Treatment Unavailable," *Times* (London), March 20, 1980, p. 4D. Nephrologists may have been perturbed, but

senior physicians in other specialties reportedly considered kidney transplantation and dialysis medical frills and believed that the funds could be used elsewhere to greater medical advantage. In the case of dialysis, the press generated enough pressure to cause the then-minister of health, John Moore, to respond in a letter acknowledging that many deaths had occurred because facilities were not available and pinpointed money as the issue. See *Sunday Mirror* (London), March 30, 1980.

23. Rodney Deitch, "Bone Marrow Transplants: Commentary from Westminster," *Lancet* 2 (December 12, 1981): 1355, as quoted in Aaron and Schwartz, *Painful Prescription,* p. 109. The *Times Health Supplement* reported later that within twenty-four hours of publication of the article, the prime minister announced a special inquiry.

Chapter Eight

1. These projections do not encompass the added costs that would be generated by extending insurance coverage to the uninsured, improving coverage for the underinsured, and closing gaps in the provision of recommended care for the well insured. Henry J. Aaron and Jack Meyer, "Health," in *Restoring Fiscal Sanity 2005: Meeting the Long-Run Challenge,* edited by Alice Rivlin and Isabel Sawhill (Brookings, 2005), pp. 73–97; Todd Gilmer and Richard Kronick, "It's the Premiums, Stupid: Projections of the Uninsured through 2013," *Health Affairs* (content.healthaffairs.org/cgi/content/full/hlthaff.w5.143/DC1 [April 5, 2005]).

2. The first step was to replace the system under which hospitals were reimbursed for costs incurred to one under which a hospital received a fixed fee for each admission. The fee is based on each patient's primary and secondary diagnoses at admission; hence the new payment method was named the diagnosis-related grouping (DRG) system. Under this system the hospital is at risk for any expenditure greater than that authorized for the particular illness; if outlays are far beyond normal, additional payments are allowed. Extra payments were made for very costly or extended stays. In addition, Medicare provided extra funds to rural hospitals, for medical training, and a variety of other special purposes.

3. When first instituted, DRG payments allowed hospitals relatively wide profit margins. Gradually meager annual adjustments squeezed out these margins. Payments for physician services were effectively restricted to meet specified targets. Congress authorized state Medicaid programs to contract with health maintenance organizations to provide services under fixed budgets.

4. Center on Medicare and Medicaid Services, *Review of Assumptions and Methods of the Medicare Trustees' Financial Projections* (Department of Health and Human Services, December, 2000).

5. John Potts and William B. Schwartz, "The Impact of the Revolution in Biomedical Research on Life Expectancy by 2050," in *Coping with Methuselah,* edited by Henry J. Aaron and William B. Schwartz (Brookings, 2004), pp. 16–51; Joseph P. Newhouse, "Medical Care Costs: How Much Welfare Loss?" *Journal of Economic Perspectives* 6, no. 3 (1992): 3–21; Aaron and Meyer, "Health."

6. For a review of several proposed ways to lower health care spending or its growth, see Aaron and Meyer, "Health."

7. See Robert Brook, "Appropriateness: The Next Frontier," *British Medical Journal* 308 (January 22, 1994): 218–19; and Albert L. Siu and others, "Inappropriate Use of Hospitals in a Randomized Trial of Health Insurance Plans," *New England Journal of Medicine* 315, no. 20 (1986): 1259–66.

8. Jonathan Skinner and John E. Wennberg, "How Much Is Enough? Efficiency and Medicare Spending in the Last Six Months of Life," Working Paper 6513 (Cambridge, Mass.: National Bureau of Economic Research, April 1998). See also John E. Wennberg, Elliott S. Fisher, and Jonathan S. Skinner, "Geography and the Debate over Medicare Reform," *Health Affairs*, web exclusive (content.healthaffairs.org/cgi/content/full/hlthaff.w2.96v1/DC1 [February 13, 2002]).

9. Lambert J.G.G. Panis, Frank W.S.M. Verheggen, and Peter Pop, "To Stay or Not to Stay. The Assessment of Appropriate Hospital Stay: A Dutch Report," *International Journal for Quality in Health Care* 14, no. 1 (2002): 55–67.

10. Oliver Sangha and others, "Metric Properties of the Appropriateness Evaluation Protocol and Predictors of Inappropriate Hospital Use in Germany: An Approach Using Longitudinal Patient Data," *International Journal for Quality in Health Care* 14, no. 6 (2002): 483–92.

11. Carles Moya-Ruiz, Salvador Peiró, and Ricard Meneu, "Effectiveness of Feedback to Physicians in Reducing Inappropriate Use of Hospitalization: A Study in a Spanish Hospital," *International Journal for Quality in Health Care* 14, no. 4 (2002): 305–12.

12. G.J. Elwyn and N.C.H. Stott, "Avoidable Referrals? Analysis of 170 Consecutive Referrals to Secondary Care," *British Medical Journal* 309 (September 3, 1994) 576–78.

13. Mark A. Schuster, Elizabeth A. McGlynn, and Robert H. Brook, "How Good Is the Quality of Health Care in the United States?" *Milbank Quarterly* 76, no. 4 (1998): 517–63.

14. Institute of Medicine, *Crossing the Quality Chasm: A New Health System for the 21st Century* (Washington: National Academy Press, 2001), p. 228

15. The reasons for the cost difference remain in dispute. One may be the age and attitudes of patients who join HMOs. Another may be the style of practice of participating physicians. Some of the savings are real and stem largely from the fact that HMOs hospitalize fewer discretionary or "unnecessary" cases than do fee-for-service providers. Nasreen Dhanani and others, "The Effect of HMOs on the Inpatient Utilization of Medicare Beneficiaries," *Health Services Research* 39, no. 5 (2004): 1607–28; Louis F. Rossiter, Lyle M. Nelson, and Killard W. Adamache, "Service Use and Costs for Medicare Beneficiaries in Risk-Based HMOs and CMPs: Some Interim Results from the National Medicare Competition Evaluation," *American Journal of Public Health* 78, no. 8 (1988): 937–43.

16. Michael Lettau, "New Statistics for Health Insurance from the National Compensation Survey," *Monthly Labor Review* 127 (August 2004): 46–50.

17. Laurence C. Baker, "Managed Care and Technology Adoption in Health Care: Evidence from Magnetic Resonance Imaging," Working Paper 8020 (Cambridge, Mass.: National Bureau of Economic Research, November 2000).

18. In addition, providing physicians financial incentives to hold down costs has been shown to reduce outlays, although evidence on the impact of such economies on the quality of care is not yet available. Martin Gaynor, James B. Rebitzer, and Lowell J. Taylor, "Physician Incentives in Health Maintenance Organizations," *Journal of Political Economy* 112, no. 4 (2004): 915–31.

19. Joseph P. Newhouse, *Pricing the Priceless: A Health Care Conundrum* (MIT, 2004). Just over one-eighth of payments to hospitals are made separately from fees set at admission for particularly lengthy or costly admissions, medical education, construction, service to patients who are uninsured, and various other functions. Jason Lee and others, "Medicare Payment Policy: Does Cost Shifting Matter?" *Health Affairs*, web exclusive (content.healthaffairs.org/cgi/content/full/hlthaff.w3.480v1/DC1 [October 8, 2003]); House of Representatives, Committee on Ways and Means, "Section 2—Medicare." *2003 Green Book*, WMCP 108-6 (Government Printing Office, March 2004).

20. Joseph Newhouse, "Reimbursing Health Plans and Health Providers: Efficiency in Production versus Selection," *Journal of Economic Literature* 34, no. 3 (1996): 1236–63.

21. Steffie Woolhandler, Terry Campbell, and David Himmelstein, "Costs of Health Care Administration in the United States and Canada," *New England Journal of Medicine* 349, no. 8 (2003): 768–75. For comments on the estimates included in the foregoing article, see Henry J. Aaron, "The Costs of Health Care Administration in the United States and Canada—Questionable Answers to a Questionable Question," *New England Journal of Medicine* 349, no. 8 (2003): 801–03.

22. This statement is based on the assumption that overall per capita health care spending continues to rise by 2.5 percentage points a year faster than income. Aaron and Meyer, "Health," pp. 89–90.

23. Gilmer and Kronick, "It's the Premiums, Stupid."

24. For details on such an approach, see Henry J. Aaron and Stuart Butler, "How Federalism Could Spur Bipartisan Action on the Uninsured," *Health Affairs*, web exclusive (content.healthaffairs.org/cgi/content/full/hlthaff.w4.168v1/DC1 [March 31, 2004]).

25. Psychological research has indicated that preferences are often poorly defined and depend on methods of elicitation. See, for example, Donald Redelmeier, Paul Rozin, and Daniel Kahneman, "Understanding Patients' Decisions: Cognitive and Emotional Perspectives," *Journal of the American Medical Association* 270, no. 1 (1993): 72–76; and Craig Fleming and others, "A Decision Analysis of Alternative Treatment Strategies for Clinically Localized Prostate Cancer," *Journal of the American Medical Association* 269, no. 20 (1993): 2650–58.

26. The recently developed left ventricular assist device is illustrative. A randomized study indicated that the device adds 7.4 months to life expectancy for the median patient at a cost of approximately $800,000 per high-quality year of survival. The service can benefit patients awaiting heart transplants and thousands of other patients with various forms of heart failure and is available from many U.S. medical centers. In 2004 the procedure was still under evaluation in Great Britain and was not generally available. On cost per quality-adjusted life year, see

Blue Cross-Blue Shield, Technical Evaluation Center, "Special Report: Cost-Effectiveness of Left-Ventricular Assist Devices as Destination Therapy for End-Stage Heart Failure," *Assessment Program* 19, no. 2 (www.bcbs.com/tec/Vol19/19_02.pdf [April 2004]). On availability in Great Britain, see British Heart Foundation, *Living with Heart Failure*, Heart Information Series no. 8 (www.bhf.org.uk/publications/uploaded/no_8.pdf [June 2005]).

27. Clifford Krauss, "In Blow to Canada's Health System, Quebec Law Is Voided," *New York Times*, June 10, 2005, p. A3.

28. Current rules governing Medigap insurance—the wraparound coverage people buy to cover copayments and deductibles charged by Medicare—illustrate clearly how *not* to handle such controls. Medicare requires patients to pay various charges for hospital and physician services. These charges are intended to limit demand for Medicare-covered services. The charges might have that effect if patients actually paid them, but most Medicare enrollees have some form of supplemental coverage that insulates them from the charges. The supplemental insurance undercuts the intended demand-reducing effects of Medicare's deductibles and copayments and boosts Medicare costs. Companies selling supplemental insurance do not pay the added costs generated within the Medicare program. By shouldering the cost of added services that such coverage engenders, taxpayers subsidize the purchase of supplemental coverage. As a result total spending is higher than what was intended by those who imposed Medicare deductibles and copayments.

29. At one time, a large proportion of CT scanners in National Health Service hospitals were donated, and some are run with private contributions. British chairs in oncology have been created by private gifts.

30. William B. Schwartz and Neal K. Komesar, "Doctors, Damages, and Deterrence: An Economic View of Medical Malpractice," *New England Journal of Medicine* 298 (June 8, 1978): 1282–89. The British definition of liability states that "the doctor will be able to defend the compensation claim successfully, if it can shown that a responsible body of reputable doctors in the relevant field would have acted in a similar manner." See Medical Negligence U.K., "Clinical Negligence Law and Compensation Claims" (www.hospitalnegligence.co.uk/clinical_negligence_definition.html [June 2005]). See also the discussion in chapter 7.

Appendix A

1. Henry J. Aaron and William B. Schwartz, *The Painful Prescription* (Brookings, 1984), p. 59.

2. Ibid., p. 138.

3. Data cited in *The Painful Prescription* fell under only two categories: total hip replacement and other arthroplasty of the hip. Presumably these two categories included revision operations, which can be performed in connection with both partial and total implants.

4. As explained in the appendix of *The Painful Prescription*, the data provided by the National Center for Health Statistics indicated that 130,367 people

received hip surgery of all kinds in 1979. This figure was increased to 145,000 to take into account the fact that some of these people will have been operated on more than once. Unlike the original statistics, the HCUP data are episode rather than person based, so it is not necessary to make this type of adjustment to the recent data. Population statistics for both years are taken from U.S. Census Bureau, *Statistical Abstract of the United States 2001*, pp. 13–14.

5. James N. Weinstein, *The Dartmouth Atlas of Musculoskeletal Health Care* (Chicago: American Hospital Association Press, 2000).

6. This figure of 71,700 is not stated explicitly in *The Painful Prescription*. It is inferred from the reported facts that 59,927 people received hip replacements in 1979, and that in 1980 about 58,500 hip replacements were performed, but that the total number of procedures was closer to 70,000 (p. 137).

7. Schurman and colleagues found that patients older than seventy-five years of age had higher rates of revision surgery than those between the ages of fifty-two and seventy-four. See D. J. Schurman and others, "Conventional Cemented Total Hip Arthroplasty: Assessment of Clinical Factors Associated with Revision for Mechanical Failure," *Clinical Orthopaedics and Related Research* 240 (March 1989): 173–80.

Index